Get Into Medical School:
A Step-by-Step Guide to the Application Process

Catherine Coleman and Lucas Nguyen

ISBN-13: 978-1508996989 ISBN-10: 1508996989

ABOUT THE AUTHORS

Catherine Coleman, fondly known as Mrs. C to her students, is a college English and ESL instructor who has been helping students improve their writing since 1999. In addition to classroom composition and language teaching, she has had the privilege of tutoring a diverse group of students, including those applying to medical school, to facilitate their scholastic goals. One of her educational endeavors has been to provide writing improvement techniques for those seeking them. Her latest project has been to help students master the medical school application process. This guide is her second publication through Coleman's Classroom, with the goal of many more to come!

Lucas Nguyen was born and raised in Vietnam. After high school, he took a year off from school, tried acting, and worked at a restaurant to experience life. Those days have given him a deep look into different life facets and have significantly formed his worldview, which is not always pink. With his family, he immigrated to the USA in 2008, immediately after which he entered Orange Coast College in Southern California, eventually transferring to UC Berkeley and graduating with the highest honor in Chemical Biology. This guide is based on his experience of applying to medical school. Currently, Lucas is pursuing his goal of becoming a physician at the University of Iowa, Carver College of Medicine.

ACKNOWLEDGMENTS

This book would not have been possible without Mr. C's continuous encouragement and willingness to give up countless weekend hours for my writing endeavors. Also, I greatly appreciate Lucas for allowing me to participate in his wild and wonderful journey of applying to medical school, which resulted in this guide to help others on the same journey. Thank you to both the Hunter and the Pirate, who are always available to listen and advise whenever I call. Finally, while there are too many to mention all by name, I must thank all those wonderful people who supported me in discussing this book, reading selections, giving feedback, and generally assisting me throughout the writing process. Specifically, thank you to my spring semester students for offering their opinions on the book's font and text size and to Nicole Bell, Christina Park, Hira Aladroos, Michelle McSkane, and Tiffany To for reading drafts and giving feedback. Also, thank you Randi Perlman for proofing the final draft! I have truly been blessed to have supportive people in my life.

For the entire process that resulted in my medical school acceptance, I would like to thank Mrs. C, who has been next to me every single step of the way to support as well as to cheer me up during the ups and downs of the application process. I would also like to thank my mom and dad, Ngoc Diep Nguyen and Phong Kien Nguyen, for wholeheartedly supporting me in pursuing my life goal. I cannot count how many times they have unconditionally fulfilled my unreasonable requests because I was so stressed. Furthermore, I would like to thank Mrs. Helen Maughan for being my second mom and always checking up on me as well as willingly helping me regardless of the day or time. I would also thank my sisters, Quynh Anh Ngoc Nguyen and Van Anh Ngoc Nguyen for teaching me new things through our interactions. Thank you, Mr. Richard Bame, for always understanding and supporting me with everything I do. Last but not least, I would like to thank all my best friends, Trevor Quach, Chau Dinh, Taryn Nguyen, Harmony Nguyen, Hang Nguyen, Vy Nguyen, Chloe Nguyen, and Phan Do Thanh Truc for always being there when I needed you. I would not be myself without all of the good influences from all of you!

CONTENTS

Timeline for Medical School Application Cycle

MARCH	MAY	JUNE	JULY	SEP	FEB	APRIL
BE READY	**PREPARE PRIMARY**	**PREPARE SECONDARY**	**PREPARE INTERVIEW**	**ATTEND INTERVIEWS**		**BE SUCCESSFUL**

Acquired	Prepare	Plan Responses	Plan	Complete	Choose
✓ MCAT	✓ Rec Letters	✓ AU	✓ Responses	✓ Practice	✓ Stress
✓ Bachelor's	✓ Essay	✓ DE	✓ Look	✓ Perform	✓ Program
✓ Volunteer	✓ Activities	✓ PA	✓ Travel		✓ Finances
✓ Research		✓ CS			✓ Environment
	Choose	✓ FP			✓ Lifestyle
	✓ Safeties	✓ SS			
	✓ Standards	✓ O			
	✓ Stretches				

CHAPTER 1: UTILIZE GUIDE

Here you are, ready to apply to medical school. You have been dreaming and planning for this experience for years. Like you, Lucas had planned his entire life on becoming a doctor. Along his journey, he enlisted the help of one of his college professors, Mrs. C. Throughout an arduous year and a half of studying, testing, writing, volunteering, working, interviewing and finally deciding, they created resources and techniques that ultimately led to Lucas' success. Currently, he is attending medical school and is on his way to achieving his dream. Given that success, Mrs. C and Lucas decided to create this guide for you, anticipating that their resources and techniques based on his experience coupled with her English expertise will assist you in achieving your dream of becoming a physician.

We have organized this guide around our medical school application cycle timeline, given in small-scale on the previous page and on a larger scale, detachable format at the end of the book. You may wish to skip around the chapters of the book based on your own needs, or you may wish to start at the beginning and go through in order. These chapters correspond to the medical school application cycle timeline to help you stay organized and on time.

Chapter 2: Be Ready is designed to help you ascertain your readiness for the medical school application process. Many students Lucas encountered along his own journey started their applications with little possibility of getting accepted because they didn't meet the minimum requirements or they were uncompetitive. If they had simply understood what was required from the beginning, they could have saved themselves many dollars, much time, and much discouragement. To avoid a similar fate, we suggest that you begin with this chapter first to make sure that you are in fact ready for the arduous application process.

The next three chapters, Chapter 3: Prepare Primary Application, Chapter 4: Prepare Secondary Application, and Chapter 5: Prepare for Interviews, are the heart of this guide with their explicit, detailed instructions for organizing and managing these stages of the application process. Though these recommendations are primarily based on our experiences so of course will not be replicated exactly in your own process, they should supply successful strategies for your application and help you avoid commonly occurring pitfalls.

Chapter 6: Prepare Alternative Routes is a chapter no one wants to read. However, statistically speaking, more than 50% of all applicants who apply to medical school the first time do not get accepted into a program. This circumstance is a very real and disheartening reality. It is our expectation that by following the guidelines here you will not be one of those unsuccessful applicants; however, there is no acceptance guarantee. You may be required to apply more than once to meet your goals. Hence, we have provided suggestions for dealing with non–admittance just in case.

One of our favorite chapters that we optimistically believe you will need to read is Chapter 7: Prepare to Succeed. Here we offer considerations for how to pick between multiple acceptances. We speak from experience in that Lucas was accepted into four medical schools and had to ultimately choose the best one for him and his future. We hope you find yourself in similar circumstances.

We wrap up our suggestions with a bit of general advice for medical school prosperity based on Lucas' first year in medical school in Chapter 8: Be Prosperous.

Ultimately, Chapter 9: Utilize Checklists and Chapter 10: Utilize Charts will be the most useful parts of this guide for your successful application. The checklists in Chapter 9 will help you stay on track and get things accomplished in a timely manner for each stage of the application process in which omitting even a single step can lead to consequent failure. Similarly, the charts in Chapter 10 provide invaluable detailed information for 134 American medical schools to help you prepare your applications. With Lucas' formula, you can expertly decide which of the schools would be the optimum selections for you based on your GPA and MCAT scores. Moreover, with the schools' previously given secondary application questions, you can prepare accomplished secondary responses. Also, you can be the most prepared for your interviews with our comprehensive, categorized interview questions. All this data has been tested in our own experiences and found to be reliable and valid for the application process.

Throughout this guide, you'll encounter a variety of specially formatted boxes to help emphasize important information. Examples of these boxes follow here.

> *Specific tips and suggestions from Mrs. C will be in the italicized Mrs. C's Tips boxes.*

Lucas' Examples from his own application process will look like this.

Questions to Ask Yourself about the various stages of the process will be indicated in this kind of box.

Interview Information will be highlighted like this.

General Charts look like this.

As a college instructor, Mrs. C has had many opportunities over the years to conference individually with students. This book attempts to provide such a one-to-one experience for you, only in written form. In taking the primary step in his medical career in his inaugural white coat ceremony at the University of Iowa, Carver College of Medicine, Lucas took the Hippocratic Oath for the first time. After years of effort and sacrifice, it was an emotionally charged moment when he swore among other things to "respect the hard-won scientific gains of those physicians in whose steps I walk, and gladly share such knowledge as is mine with those who are to follow." With this Guide, it is our intent to gladly share the knowledge we have earned through our efforts in the anticipation that you too will eventually be a physician who follows and soon takes your own Hippocratic Oath at the beginning of medical school.

Let's get started!

CHAPTER 2: BE READY
March – April

When you were preparing for and taking the MCAT, you may have believed that you were experiencing the most challenging aspect of your journey on the way to medical school. In actuality, that was only the beginning. The process itself of applying to a medical school after the MCAT is another confusing and difficult challenge that you need to conquer. The opening date for the primary application is in May, and it's important that you apply as soon as possible to be competitive against the thousands of other applicants.

Before you start preparing for your primary application, it is a good idea to ask yourself:

Am I ready for this cycle?

Answering this question positively will save you the thousands of dollars and hours of laborious writing produced from an unsuccessful application cycle. How do you ascertain if you are ready to apply? Consider the following questions to determine your readiness.

1. Are your MCAT scores and GPA sufficient?

To be eligible to submit your primary application, you must have taken the MCAT a month and a half in advance of the opening date or in advance of your application if you miss the opening date. MCAT scores are typically released 30-45 days after you take the test. Thus, taking the test as soon as possible is a priority. Although some schools will accept a primary application without the MCAT score, your file will not be reviewed by the application committee until the MCAT score is received by the school. A delay in the review could result in your application being at the end of the line for secondary and even interview consideration. For example, even if you were to submit your application one minute after the application opening time, due to a late submission of the MCAT score, your evaluation could be 1,000[th] in line. That means one thousand other candidates would have been considered before you, one thousand candidates who might have filled the opening slots for secondary applications and interviews. If the school has already chosen other applicants before your MCAT score is received and your application is reviewed, then it won't matter how high your score is or how great your application packet is — your chance of getting an interview spot will be severely hampered.

Furthermore, be realistic and evaluate whether your MCAT scores are sufficiently high enough to be considered for application. How high is high enough? This answer is not very straightforward because your MCAT score is affected by both your science class GPA and overall GPA. An MCAT score that is a little below average can be compensated for by a high GPA if your undergraduate institution has a good ranking and reputation, and vice versa, a below average GPA can be somewhat offset by a high MCAT score.

The system is currently in a transition period: starting in 2015, the MCAT was enlarged into four reorganized and expanded sections. The scoring scales for the individual tests have also changed. The MCAT Score Conversion Chart (*Chart 2: MCAT Old to New Score Conversion*) is available in Chapter 10: Utilize Charts. Prior to 2015, each of the three MCAT sections was scored on a 14-point scale from 1-15, resulting in a maximum 45 points for the total MCAT. In the new MCAT system, each of the four sections will be rated from 118-132, which is still a 14 point scale; however, the maximum score is now 528 with all four sections of the MCAT.

The average MCAT score for previously accepted medical school applicants is in the 90th percentile (32 in the OLD system or 509-510 in the NEW system), and the average overall GPA is about a 3.75. Thus, if you have a **32 MCAT OLD score (509 – 510 MCAT NEW)** and a **3.75 GPA** or above, you have a good chance of getting the golden ticket to a medical school if you pick your school wisely.

	MCAT	GPA
Sufficient Scores	32 (510 NEW)	3.75
Minimum Scores	30 (507 NEW)	3.7

What if you don't have that perfect combination?

If your MCAT is lower than a 32 OLD (509 - 510 NEW) or if your overall GPA is lower than a 3.75, the other score must be higher to compensate for the lower score. For example, according to MSAR 2014-2015, the lowest MCAT score accepted to an MD program was 28. However, that applicant probably had, at least, a 3.95 GPA to compensate for the low MCAT score, and there could have been other extenuating circumstances such as minority status or unique experiences that helped balance the low MCAT. We would not recommend applying to an MD program if you did not achieve at least a 30 OLD (507 NEW) on the MCAT regardless of your GPA. Moreover, if you didn't earn at least a 3.7 GPA both in science and overall, you probably should not apply unless you received over a 36 OLD (515 NEW) on the MCAT.

If your scores are not high enough, consider spending extra time to make your scores more competitive. To improve your MCAT score, you could retake the exam after taking an MCAT preparation class like those offered by Princeton Review or Kaplan; you could also hire a private tutor to help you study. To improve your GPA, especially your science GPA, you could take additional classes, perhaps at a community college. While there is a slim chance that you could be accepted with a marginal GPA and MCAT if your overall package is stellar, for example if you have been volunteering overseas or have published a plethora of work, it is not likely you will be accepted without sufficient scores. If you spend the time and money to apply and don't get accepted, you will need to go back and improve your scores anyway, so consider doing that before applying in the first place to save yourself the gloomy heartache, financial outlay, and time delay of not getting in.

2. Have you earned a Bachelor's degree?

Medical schools require applicants to have a Bachelor's degree or higher prior to matriculation, so make sure you meet this requirement or you will be wasting your time and money by applying. If you have an unrelated non-science graduate degree, such as an MBA, be prepared to explain why you chose a non-traditional route on the physician career path.

3. Do you have volunteer experience?

While volunteer experience is technically not a required element, it has effectively become one because the majority of applicants do meet this criterion. Thus, you should be consistently volunteering at a medical institution (e.g., hospital, clinic, urgent care facility, etc.) or a non-medical institution (e.g., nursing home, Meals on Wheels, parks, etc.) for at least six months before your application. After all, medical schools are looking for a commitment to medicine, so it doesn't make sense to state on your application that you care about the medical profession if you have not even bothered to participate in it before applying.

If you have no volunteer experience, it would be beneficial to engage in some activities during your gap year of the application cycle. Medical volunteer work would be the most appropriate, but depending on where you live, there may not be many such opportunities available to you. Check out local hospitals and nursing homes to inquire about available positions. If you are unable to find any medical-related opportunities, you can volunteer at your local library summer programs, homeless shelters, food kitchens, trash pickup, or something similar. In most American cities, the need for volunteers is much greater than the current supply.

4. Have you completed research?

This is not a required element, but since so many applicants have completed some form of research, your file will not be as competitive if you haven't. Research experience shows you can think critically. You are not going to be a full-time researcher in medical school unless you apply for an MD/Ph.D. program, so any college research you previously conducted should apply. It could be a project from any undergraduate research class, any science or social science lab internship, or even a lab job where you completed procedures on your own. If you don't have any research experience, it would be beneficial to seek some out during your gap year of medical school preparation.

5. Do you have any other relevant experience?

This category is also not expressly required, but it's an area in which you can build a unique profile to enable yourself to stand out from the highly competitive crowd. Look back on your background and see if you have any unique and relevant experiences to include in your application to make you a more diverse applicant.

Do you have any of these?

Medical Experience	MD shadowing , clinic internship, hospital internship, pharmacy internship, medical scribe, medical assistant, etc.
Leadership Experience	in clubs, honor societies, jobs, volunteer situations, etc.
Research Publications	journals, department newsletters, official publications, etc.
Academic Honors	honor societies, scholarships, academic awards, etc.
Unique Experiences	sports, debate, business, music, acting, blogging, etc.

Now that you've considered what's required to begin the application process ask yourself the following question.

Am I Ready?

Use *the Checklist 1: Readiness to Apply* in Chapter 9: Utilize Checklists to double-check your readiness for the application procedure. Review your answers to the previous five questions. If you can affirmatively respond to questions 1 and 2, and you have some experiences listed in questions 3 through 5, then you are ready for the medical school application cycle! Now you can begin the process!!!

Mrs. C's Tips: Not Worth the Gamble

If you aren't ready to apply, it's a perilous gamble. Students with deficient scores will not be accepted into medical school. Students with sufficient scores but inadequate experiences will not be accepted into medical school. This process is highly competitive, and one reason the rejection rate is so high is because many people apply before they're ready. This is probably not a worthwhile gamble to take. The application process requires an entire year; if you're not ready, you could squander that whole year. Before you start, make sure your scores and your experiences are good enough to justify the cost and the time that you will have to invest to get in! If they're not, get them ready before you begin!

CHAPTER 3: PREPARE PRIMARY APPLICATION
May – June

After ascertaining that you are ready to begin the application process, you need to consider the many steps involved in completing the primary application. Each step should be considered carefully and addressed to the best of your ability. The AMCAS application requires the following nine information sections: Identifying Information, School Information, Biographic Information, Course Work, Activity List, Letters for Evaluation, Medical School Selection, Essay, and Standardized Test Scores. Rather than simply starting with the first section and then working through each one, we have provided an alternative organizational order to maximize your efficiency. To be most effective, follow the steps in the order outlined below.

1. Open Your Application

You should start the application as soon as possible so that you can begin the other required steps. To launch the process, open the application on the AMCAS website at https://www.aamc.org, which provides clear links and videos explaining important steps in the application process. When you first open your application, you will be given an AMCAS ID, and you will choose your own username. You will also receive a confirmation email, which you should keep in case you lose or forget your information. There is no fee at this stage of the process.

2. Order Your Course Work – The Transcript

The first stage of the application review process is the transcript verification. Your application cannot be sent to any school until all your grades are verified. Schools may take weeks or even months to send out transcripts, so make sure you request your transcripts as soon as possible!

3. Request Your Letters– The Letters of Recommendation

You should request your letters of recommendation sooner rather than later. Be aware that while your application is the most important thing to you, your instructors have other priorities and may have limited ability to help you. Writing recommendation letters is an integral part of faculty members' jobs, but they do often go on vacation in the summer! Moreover, if you are asking for letters from doctors or businesses, these references may take longer than you expect. Don't be hindered in your process because you waited too long!

Also, plan carefully when collecting your letters of recommendation. You will need to make sure to have a minimum of THREE strong academic letters, which are the most important type of recommendation. Nonetheless, most schools allow you to include up to ten letters of recommendation. It is better to have more than the minimum if possible. It can be very helpful to have sources other than yourself singing your praises.

Any activity in which you have been positively involved could lead to a recommendation letter. Inarguably, medical-related activities will be the most valuable, but don't discount nonmedical-related activities as well. You are a distinctive individual with experiences differing from those of other applicants, so let your recommendation letters highlight who you are and what you are capable of. Getting into medical school requires both academic achievement and personal development; these letters offer the schools the first glimpse of why you should be admitted to their programs and how you will bring further prestige to their schools. Consider all areas of your life when planning your letters.

Mrs. C's Tips: Requesting Recommendation Letters

When you are requesting a letter from a previous instructor, make sure to include some information from that class in your request. Most instructors have taught hundreds of students, so you should not expect them to remember minute details about you. If you can, send them your personal statement or résumé. Include a picture. Help your instructors help you! It also goes without saying that you must ask promptly. Two or three weeks is a reasonable amount of time for a letter due date. Don't wait until the last minute — you may be disappointed if you do! Finally, don't forget to send a thank you card or email once the letter is received. You might need to ask that instructor for a favor in the future, so make sure to show your gratitude.

What Kind of Letters

Required Letters

You must provide THREE required letters. You must have at least TWO academic recommendations from college science instructors. Three or four would be better if possible. The best letters will come from physics, biology, or chemistry instructors. Plus, you must have at least ONE academic recommendation from a college non-science instructor. Two would be better if possible. These letters can come from any non-science class such as English, history, sociology, philosophy, or math.

Optional Letters

You may have up to SEVEN optional letters for most Medical School applications, with source suggestions listed below in the order of preferability.

1. MD with whom you have shadowed or worked for as a volunteer, scribe, medical assistant or intern for at least three months.

2. Research Publication Lead or Team Lead with whom you published a paper.

3. Supervisor in a Medical Institution where you volunteered in some capacity for at least three to six months.

4. Professor or Academic Supervisor in a Teaching Assistant Position where you taught for at least one quarter or semester.

5. Professor or Academic Supervisor in an Academic Program where you tutored or served as a lab assistant for at least one quarter or semester.

6. Supervisor in a Non-Medical location where you volunteered for at least three to six months.

7. Work Supervisor in a Non-Academic position where you have worked for at least three to six months.

8. Supervisor or Colleague in a Unique Area that may also be applied to your ability in medical school. Perhaps you have started a business, created videos, maintained an impressive blog, gone skydiving regularly, played in a band, created some new product, or completed other unique activities.

Whom to Ask For Letters

When you are asking people for letters of recommendation, many factors must be considered. Naturally, you want to ask those who will write something positive about you. In your academic classes, grades are perhaps the most important consideration, but you should also contemplate how well the professor knows you and your abilities. The length of time the person has known you is also an important factor in a letter, especially in a non-academic recommendation. Another consideration could be an outstanding effort demonstrated in some way to the letter writer. If you are asking someone to write a letter about a unique ability of yours, it would be helpful if he or she could tie this ability to your potential as a future doctor. Most people writing letters for you will be willing to tailor such letters to your specific needs, so make sure you communicate with your recommender. A final consideration is whether or not you will have access to the letter before it is sent. It is not mandatory for you to be able to read the letter; however, knowing the content will certainly help you pick and choose which letters you wish to use for certain applications. The more organized you are with the letters, the more beneficial they will be to you. You will find, in Chapter 9: Utilize Checklists, *Checklist 2: Recommendation Letters Overall* and *Checklist 3: Recommendation Letters Itemized* to help you keep track of your details.

4. Prepare Your Essay Section - The Personal Statement

Today there are many resources available to aid you in writing your personal statement. This section will offer basic advice for writing your statement based on self-reflection questions and a checklist of the information you may want to include. Your personal statement should be a snapshot of the most important things you represent with a focus on why you will be an excellent candidate for medical school.

Any actual experience you have with the medical industry should be highlighted. If you or a loved one has suffered from an illness and experienced extensive medical care, if you have worked or volunteered in the field in some way, if you have done primary research in school on a medical topic, all of these things will be important and should be emphasized. Basically, any medical experience coupled with your excellent academics should be the primary focus.

After that, consider things that make you *you*. Some examples might be socioeconomic factors, cultural or linguistic differences, unique community interests, or other personal aspects. Even as you consider other factors, always keep in mind your ultimate goal – to become a physician. Everything in your statement should lead to that explicit goal of attending medical school to become an MD.

To help you organize your ideas for your personal statement, we have broken down the brainstorming process into eight general categories of Becoming a Doctor, Acquiring Medical Experience, Earning Academic Experience, Obtaining Work Experience, Implementing Leadership Experiences, Overcoming Difficulty, Procuring Unique Experiences, and Achieving Goals. To generate ideas for your personal statement, answer as many of the questions as you can in the following box: Questions to Ask Yourself for Personal Statement.

Questions to Ask Yourself for Personal Statement

Becoming a Doctor

✓ Why do I want to be a doctor?

✓ What makes me uniquely capable of practicing medicine?

✓ What experience do I have with illness?

Acquiring Medical Experience

✓ What specific things have I done to pursue becoming a doctor?

✓ Have I volunteered, shadowed, worked in a community center, Meals on Wheels, etc.?

Earning Academic Experience

✓ Why is my GPA or MCAT score noteworthy? What awards or honors have I earned?

✓ What outstanding science experience do I have?

✓ What am I proud of? How will this help me in medical school?

Obtaining Work Experience

✓ What kind of jobs have I had?

✓ How can those experiences enable me to be successful in medical school?

Implementing Leadership and Teamwork Experiences

✓ What kind of leadership or teamwork positions have I held?

✓ What did I learn as a leader or team member that can help me to succeed in medical school?

✓ What am I proud of? How does that apply to being a doctor?

Overcoming Difficulty

✓ What problems have I had with money, family, culture, language, academics, etc.?

✓ What makes my problems unique?

✓ What did I learn that will help me become a doctor?

Procuring Unique Experiences

✓ What are my personal strengths that have led me to this point?

✓ What distinctive experiences have I had that may be relevant to my ability as a doctor?

Achieving Goals

✓ What is my long-term goal?

✓ What kind of doctor do I want to be?

✓ Where do I see myself in 10 years? In 15? In 20? How will these goals affect my being a doctor?

After generating ideas for your personal statement, you need to write those ideas in the form of an essay – this will be your personal statement. You are only allowed one page for the essay (5,300 characters with spaces), so you must be concise. The more detailed examples you can provide for the previous questions, the better your statement will be. You should plan to have only three to four main ideas, choosing from among your considered examples, which will most accurately represent your strengths. If you have overcome some meaningful adversity that has motivated you to become a doctor, such would be applicable too. Remember, the overarching question you are answering is: What makes you uniquely qualified to be admitted into medical school to become a practicing physician? In other words, you must respond to the following question:

Out of all the possible candidates,

why should a school want me?

Finally, you must consider your language and grammar usage. Excellence is never wasted, and as a physician, you will be communicating with others; in fact, your success may sometimes hinge on your ability to communicate. Long before you get to the interview and demonstrate your verbal prowess, you will be judged on your ability to communicate with the written word. That said, grammar matters. Use academic vocabulary in your statement; avoid slang and idiomatic phrases. Use complex sentences and appropriate punctuation. Have a friend read your essay to make sure that it says what you think it does. If you have the resources, have a tutor or instructor to give you suggestions. This document is one of the most important you will ever write in your life. Spend the time and effort to make it the best you can. In the following example of Lucas' personal statement, he included the previously suggested topics of Becoming a Doctor, Overcoming Difficulty, Unique Experiences, Leadership Experience, Academic Experience, Medical Experience, and Achieving Goals. It is also theme-driven as you will see the overarching theme of becoming a physician. This is just one way to write a statement; in actuality, there are many useful ways. Remember, the key is that you identify your unique abilities and explain why becoming a physician is vital for you. Convince your reader that you, above all others, should go to that school. Use *Checklist 4: Personal Statement* in Chapter 9: Utilize Checklists to help you create your own personal statement.

Mrs. C's Tips: Using Examples

Reading examples provides both advantages and disadvantages. On the one hand, good examples can provide ideas and inspiration; on the other hand, even good examples can be limiting if you try to match the format or content exactly. With the examples in this book, an effective strategy of usage would be to note what aspects of the example you find relevant to your life or experience. Then you can customize your own response based on the general ideas or vocabulary provided. I can't stress enough the importance of NOT merely copying a section from an example. In an academic environment, copying is called cheating or more precisely plagiarism. I can't think of any faster way to get denied acceptance to a medical school than cheating in an attempt to get in.

	Lucas' Personal Statement
Questions Answered	*bolded phrases relate to questions answered

Becoming Doctor Procuring Unique Experiences

Though neither of my parents completed high school in Vietnam, they recognized my potential and encouraged me to pursue a medical career believing this would shape me into a compassionate person. As a youth, I followed my parents' guidance without thinking about why I wanted to become a doctor, **simply studying because I was good at it**. Five years ago, after I finished high school, my family immigrated to America. A week after arriving, I started community college despite having little English vocabulary and facing cultural shock because of this language barrier. However, I overcame this difficulty by maximizing my communication with people around me and excelled in all my classes, **so I continued to pursue the medical dream**.

Overcoming Difficulty

During my first year of college, my mom, in financially supporting the family, **contracted hepatitis C** in her job as a permanent make-up artist, and through her sickness and journey toward health, **I discovered my own desire to become a doctor.** As part of my mom's treatment, her self-injections of alpha interferons combined with ribavirin caused severe side effects and a low red blood cell count. For her first blood test result, my mom asked me to drive her to the doctor's office, but deprived of sleep because of school and work, I refused. As she got in the car, the anxiety of getting the result coupled with her chronic asthma induced a panic attack, causing her to pass out. When the paramedics came, and I observed them taking care of her, I realized that doctors do not simply **prescribe medicine, but actually, they provide patient care**. It was at that moment I finally realized exactly **why I want to be a doctor: I want to care for others.**

Becoming Doctor

After that day, I was by my mom's side through everything. I researched her disease's side effects, spoke with her doctor, comforted her, monitored her medications, and gave her weekly injections. Her sickness slowly got better, and **I became a healer.** When the doctor told my mom she was cured, she glowed, and as she gave him a hug, the doctor glowed as well. **Through that cathartic moment becoming a doctor had now become my dream, not just my parents'.** With this new purpose for medical practice, my interest in medicine escalated to the next level.

I became an advocate and spread my passion to many people around me through my leadership activities. I regularly participated in my community college's annual Science Night, **leading a group of students** to perform chemistry demonstrations for children to encourage their interest in science. To motivate even more children, the team made a YouTube channel called Chemistry Kicks Acid, posting easy-to-do at-home chemistry experiments. Plus, **I invented a tool called Chemplate** for drawing organic molecules to help chemistry students with their homework. I founded the Chemplate Company and have sold the Chemplates in many bookstores, universities, and lab companies. Because the Chemplate makes homework easier, it increases students' interest in chemistry. Then, as an undergraduate student instructor at UC Berkeley, when **I included real life applications in my pre-lab talks**, some students were so fascinated by this information they decided to major in the health field. **My passion to serve others in medicine grew** with each activity, and seeing people gain interest in medicine made me feel rewarded.

Moreover, majoring in chemical biology played a major role in preparing me for the medical field. In addition to taking classes, working in the chemistry department lab at Orange Coast College exposed me to situations that improved my **critical thinking and problem-solving skills**. After transferring to UC Berkeley, my multiple scholarships enabled me to not work, **focusing only on school and thriving in the immense knowledge and research opportunities**. There, in a research lab class, I studied RNA regulation and immersed myself in the art of independent and group study. Being constantly exposed to the critical thinking process has solidified my knowledge as well as prepared me for the upcoming heavy course load in medical school, and with a clear goal and aspiration to spread my passion, I believe that I am ready to take my education to the next level to achieve my career goal, not only as a doctor but also as a healer.

Inspired by this goal, **I joined several volunteer organizations** to enrich my passion for healing. At UC **Irvine Medical Center**, through interactions with patients, I was able to listen to their needs and learn what they expect from their doctors. I also learned about the organization of the hospital, about interdepartmental interactions, and about diseases prevention during an epidemic. Simultaneously, while **interning at a clinic**, I learned about the daily life of a doctor through shadowing Dr. Wong. He also taught me about the healthcare system and the business aspect of a medical practice. With Dr. Wong, **I traveled to treat the ill in Vietnam**, performing patient care in rural communities. **As I volunteered,** I was constantly reminded the most rewarding thing for a doctor is his patients' health. I know as a medical student and ultimately a doctor, I will have intense pressure from school and the job; however, as I immerse myself in the pursuit of patients' wellness, **I will maintain my motivation to heal**.

Mrs. C's Tips: Writing the Personal Statement

❖ *Use Action Verbs!*

When writing about your experiences, you will be extremely limited in your word count, so using powerful action verbs like the ones below will help you get your ideas across. Make sure the verb is the appropriate one for the specific action and use a variety of verbs. For example, if you volunteered in a hospital as a reception greeter, then you could use other verbs, like contributed, assisted, or supported, to explain the experience. For example:

- o *contributed to the hospital environment as a reception greeter*
- o *assisted, aided, or helped the hospital as a greeter*
- o *offered helpful information to people as a hospital greeter*
- o *supported the overall hospital information system as a greeter*
- o *facilitated communication within the hospital as a greeter*
- o *promoted good communication in a hospital as a reception greeter*

When writing your personal statement, use a variety of specific action verbs like the ones below.

	Acquire	*Conquer*	*Guide*	*Offer*	*Succeed*
	Administer	*Direct*	*Help*	*Obtain*	*Supervise*
Action	*Aid*	*Dispense*	*Improve*	*Overcome*	*Support*
Verbs	*Assist*	*Earn*	*Inspire*	*Prevail*	*Teach*
	Benefit	*Energize*	*Maintain*	*Profit*	*Train*
	Coach	*Facilitate*	*Master*	*Promote*	*Volunteer*
	Contribute	*Gain*	*Mentor*	*Serve*	*Win*

❖ *Use Active and Passive Voice!*

Don't be afraid to use both active and passive voice. Using both can reveal a strong sense of academic ability as well as make your personal statement stand out from others. While you may have earned a 4.0 GPA at Berkeley or obtained a spectacular MCAT score, perhaps your desire to be a physician was energized through your volunteer work in a clinic or a difficulty was overcome through your perseverance.

❖ *Use Descriptive Adjectives*

Make sure you are using the correct adjective and that it is a meaningful one. If none of the adjectives given below meet your needs, don't hesitate to use a good college thesaurus!

	Advantageous	Consequential	Injurious	Educational
	Beneficial	Eventful	Harmful	Informational
Descriptive	Favorable	Momentous	Unfavorable	Enlightening
Adjectives	Promising	Significant	Unhelpful	Comprehensive
	Desirable	Central	Disadvantageous	Scholarly
	Supportive	Crucial	Adverse	Constructive

❖ *Use the First Person Singular point of view as much as possible.*

This is the section for you to genuinely show why you are special and should be admitted, so avoid using "we" and "our" as much as possible. Even if you were on a team project, you could use "I as a team leader," or "I as team contributor" rather than "we the team." Of course, you can use the plural 1st person "we" or 3rd person "they", but as much as possible focus on I, me, my, and myself. You are the one applying for entrance, not your team.

❖ *Use Appropriate Transitions*

Many writers often use the same worn out transitions like "on the other hand" and "nowadays." Even worse, they begin sentences with coordinate conjunctions like "but" or "and." Stand out from the rest of the applicants by using the better and more appropriate transitions below to help your personal statement flow.

INSTEAD OF		USE	
And	Additionally	Moreover	Plus
But	Conversely	In Contrast	Nevertheless
For Example	Likewise	Similarly	Particularly

5. Prepare Your Activity List –Personal Experiences

The Activity List section of the application will allow you to list a maximum of fifteen activities with a very brief experience description (700 characters with spaces). You will also have three paragraphs (1325 characters with spaces) to discuss the most meaningful activities. You have already considered these experiences as you brainstormed your ideas for the personal statement. However, here you have the opportunity to include many more experiences than in the personal statement. No significant experience is too small for your initial consideration. Try and brainstorm at least twenty and then you can pick the fifteen most applicable for the medical school application. Go back and revisit the questions from your personal statement. Is there any experience you left out? Some possible activities for your General Experiences Activity List could be:

Medical Activities	Academic Activities	Extracurricular Activities
Physician Shadow	Research	Team Leader
Medical Assistant	Awards	Team Member
Physician Scribe	TA	General Volunteer
Medical Intern	Peer Tutor	Club Member
Medical Volunteer	Science Lab	Musician

What kinds of activities have you completed?

Within these broad categories, you might have had multiple experiences. For instance, perhaps you volunteered in both a hospital and a clinic. How were those experiences different? What have you learned from both? Or maybe you overcame both financial and physical hardship. Both those experiences would have taught you distinctive lessons that can be applied to medical school.

You will need to sort your experiences into these eighteen categories: Artistic, Athletics, Conferences, Extracurricular, Hobbies, Honors, Leadership, Military, Paid-Medical, Paid-Nonmedical, Presentation/Posters, Publications, Other, Research, Shadowing, Teaching, Volunteer-Medical, and Volunteer-Nonmedical. Be aware that not all categories are equally valued by acceptance committees. Any medical experience is more relevant than other experiences. It may not be possible to fulfill all eighteen categories, but try your best to do so as much as possible to have a spectrum of experiences to show your well-rounded capabilities. It is not necessary to order the importance as the submission process will automatically alphabetize your entries.

Review two of Lucas' Experience Description Examples given below. The first (Shadowing a Physician) is 698 characters and the second (Volunteering-Nonmedical) is 473. Both models explain the experience and show its relevance, whether explicit in the first or implied in the second. As always, remember that examples are just that – examples. They are not meant to provide rules or obligations for your own experiences.

Lucas' Experience Description

Shadowing Physician

During my surgical shadowing experience at the Quant Y 7A Hospital in Ho Chi Minh City, Viet Nam, I observed several surgical procedures from anesthetization to recovery. Moreover, I was exposed to the different techniques of intubating a patient, inserting an IV, and changing a patient's position. Simultaneously, while the surgeons were operating, they discussed with me the surgical techniques of the case. In the orthopedic tendon connection case, the surgeon instructed me on the pros and cons of different types of sutures and their usages to achieve the best result. I now understand being a surgeon requires great responsibility and tremendous effort as well as compassion for the patients.

Volunteering Non-Medical

For three years, I have participated in Orange Coast College's annual Science Night, in which all the departments have an open house and perform interesting demonstrations for children. The chemistry department, of which I am a part, presents a variety of experiments such as fireworks with various metals. Moreover, I have led a group of students in performing easy-to-do-at-home chemistry experiments, like making lava lamps, to develop the children's interest in science.

You are not required to have all fifteen activities filled out; however, the more experience you provide related to your goal, the more competitive you will be in the admissions process. As you think about your experiences, try to link them to qualities of successful students. Of the fifteen allowed activities, twelve of them are very brief (only 700 characters with spaces), so be concise!

Once you have chosen your fifteen experiences, choose the three experiences that are most applicable to medicine and your career goals for your three most meaningful paragraphs. Explain the aspects of the experience that will benefit you as a medical student or practicing physician. The activity section requires both Experience Description and Experience Remarks, which is where you explain the importance of the experience. As you review Lucas' two given examples, note that only one is related to medicine under Paid Medical; the second one is under is Tutoring/Teaching, which relates to academic success. The goal is to show how the particular event will contribute to future achievements in medical school.

Lucas' Most Meaningful Activities

[Experience Description]
As an intern in the Joshua Medical Group, I started with patient outreach, leading other volunteers to organize multiple activities at senior homes to encourage healthy lifestyles and build their relationships with the clinic. I also helped organize the clinic's senior health fair. Plus, I performed patient observations and surveys to help the clinic run smoothly and reduce the patient wait time. With Dr. Wong, I studied the healthcare system as well as the business aspects of a medical practice. Also, as the clinic is expanding toward an Accountable Care Organization, I have joined a team to improve the clinic's quality measure report to increase its ranking during certification.

[Experience Remarks]
Interning at the Joshua Medical Group has provided me with multiple opportunities to grow as a person and widen my view about the role of a physician. With seniors, especially those with Alzheimer's, I learned to be patient in their arts and crafts instruction. I also learned to follow through with their weekly activity requests. Through these little lessons and as my maturity and responsibility grew, I could see the seniors increasingly benefited since the quality of our time improved significantly. Ultimately, seeing them become more positive has motivated me to perform future patient outreach. Moreover, my time at the clinic has given me a better idea about a physician's role. Through observation, I discovered that besides examining and prescribing patients with medications, a doctor has to deal with insurance companies while balancing between his definition of patients' wellness and government regulations. On top of that, he has to make sure that the clinic generates enough income to sustain the business and secure the employees' jobs. Thus, as I assumed different positions within the clinic, I finally sensed the amount of stress that is pushing down on the physician's shoulders. This experience has trained me to multitask more efficiently and prepared me for the amount of work waiting ahead.

Interning In Medical Environment

Teaching / Tutoring

[Experience Description]

At UC Berkeley, as an undergraduate student instructor for organic chemistry, I facilitated student learning in both lecture and lab sections for two semesters. In the lecture sections, I assisted students by holding weekly office hours and review sessions, grading midterms, and final exams, and advising with strategies to excel in the class. In the lab sections, I prepared weekly pre-lab talks, helped students troubleshoot during experiments, ensured lab safety, set up a lab report format, graded students' work, and wrote recommendation letters upon request. My goal was to make sure that the students retained basic information as well as were treated equally to maintain fairness.

[Experience Remarks]

Through teaching, I grew academically because explaining the class materials both solidified and widened my content knowledge when the students posed questions that I had never previously considered forcing me to do my own research to find satisfactory answers. More importantly, I matured through this experience as I was constantly advising students in labs about techniques, time management, or how to work in groups. My leadership skills have improved significantly since I had to simultaneously monitor 30 people. Also, because of my direct responsibility for the students' grades, I faced multiple ethical dilemmas and learned to set aside my emotion and only formulate grades rationally. Ultimately, these experiences have catalyzed my efforts to become a well-rounded individual. I also noticed a transformation in many students. My attempts to include pragmatic information about the medical field in my pre-lab talks made learning more interesting and engaged the students in chemistry. As a result, many of them completed the class with high grades, and some actually thought about changing their majors to a health field. Moreover, as a strict teacher, my enforcement of discipline in class caused many students to report they learned to take their schoolwork more seriously.

There is also a section in the application to discuss any disadvantages you may have encountered in your life. This section is where you can discuss any financial hardship you may have experienced that may affect you in medical school. If this applies to you, make sure you have a detailed paragraph to explain the situation. Make sure that if you do explain a disadvantage, that it is a valid one, something unique that not everyone striving for medical school has likely encountered.

6. Choose Your Medical Schools - The Best Fit

When deciding which schools to apply for, you have to consider many possible qualifications. Some applicants prefer particular environments or weather conditions. Some people are not willing to move out-of-state. Others decide based on school ranking for a research or primary care path. Cost may be a very real consideration as well.

While all these factors may play a role in your decision, we suggest you choose your schools primarily on what you qualify for based on the THREE FACTORS of out-of-state acceptance rates, MCAT scores, and GPA. Included in Chapter 10: Utilize Charts, *Chart 4: School Selection Statistics*, is a list of 134 American medical schools' 2014 information scores to help you gauge which schools you best qualify for. We recommend that you apply to a total of 30-40 schools to assure a spot in an MD program next year, and it is important to choose the schools where you have the best chance of acceptance. How can you rationally decide? Some factors can't be planned for such as the popularity of a location. Nevertheless, in making your school choice, you should consider two main factors: State Residency and Scores. Following these guidelines will help you select the most favorable options.

Choosing Appropriate State Residency

The first thing to do is look at the school's residency requirements. It doesn't matter how much you want to attend a school or what your scores are if you do not meet that fundamental prerequisite. Many schools only accept in-state students or very few out-of-state students. Thus, just because of the circumstances of your state residency, applying to schools that limit residency could be disadvantageous for you. Therefore, the first thing you should do is plan to apply to all the schools that are in your state-of-residence. Even if you live in a large state with multiple schools, like California or Texas, plan to apply to all the schools in your state. You may have an advantage in your own state compared to out-of-state applicants.

Then use *Chart 4: School Selection Statistics* in Chapter 10: Utilize Charts to identify which other schools are actually available to you. Note all of the schools that are marked with a **YES** in the In-State column; this yes means the school either requires in-state residency or prefers it. If you are not currently living in one of those states, you will have less of a chance of admission to those schools. By choosing schools that are marked with a **NO** in the In-State column, you will have the best chance for acceptance.

Choosing Appropriate Schools

A favorable strategy for getting into medical school is to choose schools for which your scores place in the median of previously accepted applicants' scores. If your scores are too high, then schools may think you will get better offers from higher-ranked schools, so they may not accept you despite your excellent scores. Also, if your scores are too low, then others who have higher scores may be chosen first, eliminating you completely or causing you to be waitlisted. Remember, every school has a limited number of available student positions to fill. Thus, choosing schools for which you are the best fit will facilitate your acceptance. We have organized schools into five categories: STANDARD, SAFETY, STRETCH, UNSUITABLE, AND UNCLEAR.

For your first choices, STANDARD schools should make up the majority of your selections as those are the places where you will have the best chance of acceptance. You can also have some SAFETY schools and a few STRETCH schools as well. Overall, to give yourself the best chance of securing acceptance, you will want to choose a total of around forty schools: twenty to thirty STANDARD schools, five SAFETY schools, and five STRETCH schools. You can vary the numbers as you wish, but the bulk of your school selections should be in the STANDARD range to give you the best chance of acceptance.

To best match your MCAT score and GPA to the schools' normal ranges, look at each school's previously reported data tabulated in *Chart 4: School Selection Statistics* in Chapter 10: Utilize Charts. For each school, the MCAT (OLD) column provides the low / median/ high ranges of the previously accepted students' scores, and the MCAT (NEW) column has the conversion numbers for the MCAT scores as of 2015 although the data for students' acceptance rates is not yet available. Similarly, both columns of GPA ALL, which is the overall GPA, and GPA S, which is the overall science GPA, provide the same low / median /high range data. Consider the example following MCAT and GPA example charts.

MCAT (OLD)		27	33	37	
School Score Range		(low)	(median)	(high)	
MCAT (NEW)	UNSUITABLE	502-503 ⟷	511	⟷ 516-517	UNSUITABLE
School Score Range		(low)	(median)	(high)	
Your MCAT Score		**STRETCH School**	**STANDARD School**	**SAFETY School**	

Your GPA	UNSUITABLE	STRETCH School	STANDARD School	SAFETY School	UNSUITABLE
GPA ALL School Score Range		3.37 (low)	3.72 (median)	3.95 (high)	
GPA S School Score Range		3.27 (low)	3.69 (median)	3.98 (high)	

- ✓ STRETCH schools are those for which your MCAT score and GPA rank from the lowest to the median score.
- ✓ STANDARD schools are those for which your MCAT score and GPA rank at the median.
- ✓ SAFETY schools are those for which your MCAT score and GPA rank from the median to the highest score.
- ✓ UNSUITABLE schools are those for which your MCAT and GPA either rank below the lowest score or above the highest score.

Usually, a typical student's MCAT score will be directly proportional to the GPA. Thus, if you have scored in the 90th percentile for the MCAT (33 OLD or 512 NEW), your overall GPA should be around 3.75, also in the 90th percentile. If your scores correlate in this way, your tasks are relatively straightforward. However, sometimes scores do not correlate so neatly, and in that case, you'll have to do some extra work because your scores are UNCLEAR. A UNCLEAR school is one for which your MCAT score is at one level, and your GPA is at another. In that case, you want to use the higher of the scores to evaluate where you fit in a school's ranking. If you have a high MCAT score but a low GPA, you can use the higher one to compensate for the lower. For example, if your MCAT is lower than the median school score but your GPA ALL is at the median or higher, you can choose the higher GPA ranges in the GPA columns. In the same way, a high MCAT score can compensate for a lower GPA, so use the MCAT score to choose your schools.

Mrs. C's Tips: Special Exception!

If you belong to a medically underrepresented minority group such as African American, Native American, or Mexican American, you can apply to schools with a slightly higher median in both MCAT and GPA (about 2-3 points for MCAT and 0.2-0.3 for GPA). The strong demand for diversity in many medical schools may give you a more competitive edge!

Choosing Appropriate Schools		
School Type	MCAT	GPA
STRETCH	Your MCAT score is between the school's lowest score and the median.	Your GPA is between the school's lowest score and the median.
STANDARD	Your MCAT score is equal to the school's median score.	Your GPA is equal to the school's median score.
SAFETY	Your MCAT score is between the school's median and the highest score.	Your GPA is between the school's median and the highest GPA.
UNSUITABLE	Your MCAT score is below the school's lowest score or above the highest score.	Your GPA is below the school's lowest score or above the highest score.
UNCLEAR	Your MCAT score and GPA don't correlate causing a discrepancy in ranking possibilities. Usually match the higher possibility that to a school's scores.	

Choosing STANDARD schools

This category of schools should make up the majority of your choices. We suggest you apply to twenty to thirty STANDARD schools. To do so, after eliminating all the schools from Step 1, look at the MCAT and GPA median scores for the schools to which you qualify. You want to choose schools for which your scores place exactly at the median. For instance, if a school's MCAT scores are 27 / 33 / 37 (OLD) or 502 - 503 / 511 / 516 - 517 (NEW) and your MCAT score is 33 (505 - 506 NEW), then this school would be a STANDARD school for you. Initially consider the MCAT score as weightier than the GPA score as you review the data, but do use the higher of your two scores. Also, if your unevenly correlated scores cause you to have UNCLEAR schools, use the greater number of the MCAT score or GPA to choose your schools.

Choosing SAFETY Schools

SAFETY schools also provide a good probability of acceptance, so now choose five additional schools for which your scores place between the median and the highest score. For these schools, you will be above their median average so you will be their best choice! Just remember, don't go too low or you might end up waitlisted instead. For the previous example school range, four MCAT scores would place into the SAFETY category.

MCAT Score Range	27 / 33 / 37 (OLD) 502 – 503 / 511 / 516 – 517 (NEW)	
Your MCAT	34 (512 – 513)	35 (514)
	36 (515)	37 (517)

Choosing STRETCH schools

While the majority of your school choices should consist of schools for which you have a better chance of being accepted, go ahead and reach for the top and choose five STRETCH schools if you like. You have been striving to get to this place your entire college career thus far; don't limit yourself. You never know whether or not a school may take an interest in you. This could also be a place to include schools that had a YES for In-State. But don't pin much hope on your STRETCH schools as they will be chancy in terms of acceptance

For these schools, you will be below their median average, which means a large number of students will have scored higher than you. Based on your scores alone, you will not be competitive. Nevertheless, you may have other aspects of your application packet such as your experience or background that allow you to have a chance at a STRETCH school.

For previously given example school range, six MCAT scores would place into the STRETCH category.

MCAT Score Range	27 / 33 / 37 (OLD) 502 – 503 / 511 / 516 – 517 (NEW)		
Your MCAT	27 (502 – 503)	28 (504)	29 (505-506)
	30 (507)	31 (508)	32 (509 – 510)

Avoiding UNSUITABLE schools

These are schools for which your scores really don't qualify at all; therefore, you have a very minuscule chance of getting accepted. One of the reasons the non-acceptance rate is so high for medical school is that students apply to schools for which they just don't have the scores to get in. If your MCAT score and GPA are below a school's lowest score, this school would be a UNSUITABLE school for you. Also, if your MCAT score and GPA are above a school's highest score, that school is UNSUITABLE. While it might seem reasonable that schools would want you more if your scores are significantly higher than the general student population, this is actually not the case. In actuality, having too high of a score is just as detrimental as having a score that is too low. We do not suggest that you apply to any UNSUITABLE schools.

MCAT Score Range	27 / 33 / 37 (OLD) 502 – 503 / 511 / 516-517 (NEW)		
Your MCAT	TOO LOW		
	5-10 (472 - 479)	11-20 (480 - 493)	21-26 (494 - 501)
	TOO HIGH		
	38-40 (518 - 521)		41-45 (522 - 528)

Identifying UNCLEAR schools

Furthermore, it may be difficult to categorize some schools if you have atypical or uneven scores. If you have a particularly high 3.9 GPA but only an average 33 MCAT score, it will make it harder to distinguish between STANDARD, SAFETY, and STRETCH schools. With UNCLEAR schools, you'll have to decide on a case-by-case basis. Generally speaking, you want to choose the higher level unless it's so high as to be unsuitable.

Once you have selected your schools, make sure you have chosen a variety of schools. As you discover which schools you qualify for, you might want to rank them to make sure that you apply to the schools where you will be the most competitive first, and then to the other schools where you may be less competitive. Use *Checklist 5: My School Choices* and *Checklist 6 School Selection Overall:* in Chapter 9: Utilize Checklists to help you with the details.

Mrs. C's Tips: Guidelines Not Rules

This formula is a general guideline, not a precise rule. You may find that your scores are more unclear than exact, especially for the STANDARD scores. Don't get stressed if this happens. Just choose your best scores that accurately represent your proven abilities. Lucas had a similar problem. His 4.0 GPA ALL and S were at the top, but his 34 MCAT score wasn't quite as high creating a discrepancy that had to be juggled. If you find that your scores do not match, or you have difficulty choosing STANDARD schools, make sure to choose more SAFETY schools than STRETCH. With the STANDARD and SAFETY schools, you have a good chance to get into the school as your scores are competitive. With the STRETCH, you have less of a chance, maybe none at all. If you choose mostly schools for which you are not competitive, then you will be redoing this process next year. Remember, getting in means applying where you qualify to go, not just where you want to go!

Understand the School Selection Process

The examples and excerpt from *Chart 4: School Selection Statistics* for the University of Washington illustrate how to use this data.

#	School				
	MCAT (OLD)	MCAT (NEW)	GPA ALL	GPA S	In-State
123	**University of Washington**				
	27 / 31 / 38	502 - 503 / 508 / 518	3.4 / 3.73 / 3.97	3.2 / 3.69 / 3.98	N

STANDARD Score - MCAT 31 (508); GPA ALL 3.73

The 31 (508) MCAT score places at the school median 31 MCAT score and the 3.73 GPA ALL at the school median 3.73 GPA ALL making this a STANDARD school.

UNCLEAR Score – High MCAT / Low GPA: MCAT 32 (509 - 510); GPA ALL 3.5

The 32 (509-510) MCAT score places above the school median 31 MCAT score making this a SAFETY school; the 3.5 GPA ALL places between the school low 3.4 and median 3.73 GPA ALL making it a STRETCH school. Averaging the two, makes this school a STANDARD school.

UNCLEAR Score – MCAT 30 (507); GPA ALL 3.75; GPA S 3.69

The 30 (507) MCAT score places below the school median 31 MCAT score making this a STRETCH school; the 3.75 GPA ALL places just slightly above the school median 3.73 GPA ALL making this a SAFETY school; the 3.69 GPA S places at the school median 3.69 GPA S, making this a STANDARD school. Averaging the three, makes this school a STANDARD school.

SAFETY Score: MCAT 35 (508); GPA ALL 3.85

The 35 (508) MCAT score places between the school median 31 and high 38 MCAT scores and the 3.85 GPA ALL also places between the school median 3.73 and high 3.97 GPA ALL scores making this a SAFETY school.

STRETCH Score: MCAT 29 (505 - 506); GPA ALL 3.6

The 29 (505-506) MCAT score places between the school low 27 and median 31 MCAT scores, and the 3.6 GPA ALL places between the school low 3.4 and median 3.73 GPA ALL making this a STRETCH school.

UNSUITABLE Score MCAT 24 (498 - 499); GPA ALL 3.3

The 24 (498-499) MCAT score places below the school low 27 MCAT score and the 3.3 GPA ALL places below the 3.4 GPA ALL making this a UNSUITABLE school.

Double Check Your Understanding

Let's look at some real scenarios with three Californian applicants' scores. Fill in the appropriate school choices for each applicant based on their MCAT scores, overall GPA, and the school information chart excerpt from *Chart 4: School Selection Statistics* to deduce where they should apply.

	MCAT	GPA	SAFETY	STANDARD	STRETCH
Julia	34	3.73			
Alex	33	3.6			
Sam	30	3.59			

#	School				
	MCAT (OLD)	MCAT (NEW)	GPA ALL	GPA S	In-state
5	**Brown (Warren Alpert)**				
	28 / 33 / 37	504 / 511 / 516-517	3.41/3.75/3.96	3.2/3.73/3.99	N
23	**Harvard**				
	32 / 37 / 41	509-510 / 516-517 / 522	3.73 / 3.93 / 4	3.73 / 3.94 / 4	N
38	**Meharry Medical College**				
	24 / 27 / 30	498 - 499 / 502-503 / 507	3.2 / 3.52 / 3.88	3.03 / 3.41 / 3.88	N
51	**Quinnipiac University (Netter)**				
	27 / 30 / 34	502-503 / 507 / 512-513	3.28 / 3.59 / 3.86	3.15 / 3.53 / 3.88	N
68	**Tulane**				
	31 / 33 / 36	508 / 511 / 515	3.27 / 3.61 / 3.9	3.12 / 3.51 / 3.91	N
71	**Tufts**				
	30 / 34 / 38	507 / 512- 513 / 518	3.42 / 3.73 / 3.94	3.31 / 3.7 / 3.96	N

With her 34 MCAT and 3.73 GPA, **Julia's schools** are:

SAFETY	Tulane with her 34 MCAT placing between its median 33 and high 36 MCAT score and her 3.73 GPA placing between its median 3.61 and high 3.9 GPA. Netter with her 34 MCAT placing between its median 30 and high 34 MCAT score and her 3.73 GPA placing between its median 3.59 and high 3.86 GPA.
STANDARD	Tufts with her 34 MCAT score and 3.73 GPA placing her firmly in the median.
STRETCH	Harvard with her 34 MCAT placing between its low 32 and median 37 MCAT score and her 3.73 GPA placing between its low 3.73 and high GPA.

With his 33 MCAT and 3.6 GPA, **Alex's schools** are:

SAFETY	Netter with his 33 MCAT placing between its median 30 and high 34 MCAT score and his 3.6 GPA placing between its median 3.59 and high 3.86 GPA.
STANDARD	Tulane with his 33 MCAT and his 3. 6 GPA placing him firmly in the median.
UNCLEAR	Brown with his 33 MCAT score placing at its median 33 MCAT score making it STANDARD school; his 3.6 GPA placing between its low 3.41 and median 3.75 making it a STRETCH school.
UNSUITABLE:	Harvard with his 33 MCAT placing between its low 32 and median 37 MCAT score and his 3.6 GPA placing below the low 3.73 GPA making it a UNSUITABLE school.

With his 30 MCAT and 3.59 GPA, **Sam's schools** are:

SAFETY	Meharry with his 30 MCAT placing between its median 27 and high 30 MCAT score and his 3.59 GPA placing between median its 3.52 and high 3.88 GPA.
STANDARD	Netter with his 30 MCAT and 3.59 GPA placing him firmly in the median.
STRETCH	Brown with his 30 MCAT placing between its low 28 and median 33 MCAT score and his 3.59 GPA placing between its low 3.41 and high 3.75 GPA.

7. Complete Application Sections – The Details

Having completed the most time-consuming aspects of the application, you can now update your application with the rest of the sections: standardized test, ID information, schools attended information, and biographic information. Make sure that you are careful when inputting the information as errors can cause delays in the process. Also, consider the following factors for your application:

✓ Contact Information.

It is a good idea to have a formal email like your first initial and last name, i.e. ccoleman@clmn.net, rather than something fun you might already be using like eslteachersrock@gmail.com. Consider creating an appropriate email account name if you don't already have one. You also might consider creating a mailbox just for the application process so you don't miss an important communication that got buried among other emails in your crowded inbox!

✓ Disadvantaged Information

Any cultural, linguistic, or financial disadvantages you have encountered that may affect your application process may be included on the application. Just like for your experiences, you should have already prepared these compelling, well-written specific examples in a paragraph while working on the experience section of the process – if you haven't, do so now!

✓ Patience.

You will need to have many specific details and much patience for the 17 to 20 page application. It may be easier for you to have some of this information typed already so you can copy and paste. Make sure you have verified the correctness of all the data. You don't want your application stalled in admissions due to a typo! Also, you don't have to complete it all at once, so if you find yourself getting overwhelmed, take a break and come back later when you are refreshed.

✓ Verification.

Before you hit the final submit button, verify all your data. Make sure there are no typos or misremembered information. This is an important step, so don't omit it!

8. Relax!

Whew! You have done it! The primary application is submitted. Take a deep breath and congratulate yourself for a job well done. Maybe, take a day or even two off.

Then, however, gear up and start preparing for the next stage, the secondary applications! The next chapter will help you prepare for that step of the process.

CHAPTER 4: PREPARE SECONDARY APPLICATION
June-August

After you have submitted the primary application, you will have to wait for the schools to send secondary application requests, but you should not be idle during this time. To make the best use of your time, you can prepare your responses to possible questions. Not only can you create responses to general questions, but also you can look at the school's previously asked secondary application questions. If you applied to multiple schools as we suggested, then many secondary application requests will come in at the same time. In any given week during his application cycle, Lucas received as many as four secondary application requests. Throughout the process, he was juggling six to eight secondary applications at the same time. The key to his success in managing these secondary responses in a timely manner was preparation and organization. If you don't do well in the secondary applications, you will not be offered interviews.

After an extensive review of the secondary questions used in the 2014-2015 application cycle, we have categorized seven general topics that you can prepare for. These topics are Autobiographical / Uniqueness (AU), Diversity Experiences (DE), Challenging Situations (CS), School Specific (SS), Future Plans (FP), and Other Topics (O). The secondary questions from 2014-2015 are listed in the Appendices, *Chart 6: Secondary Application Questions*. While it is a good idea to review the questions for your particular schools, there are absolutely no guarantees that the exact same questions will be asked during your secondary application cycle. Thus, rather than answering the specific questions, it is a more practical and efficient strategy to write general answers to each of the category topics, which are explained in greater detail in this chapter. Let's explore each of these categories.

Explore the Categories

Autobiographical / Uniqueness – AU

The autobiographical questions seek answers about who you are, what you have done, and why you want to practice medicine. A few schools ask for an actual autobiography or chronology of your life. Other schools ask questions about what kind of research you have conducted or what extra-curricular activities you have been involved in. Of course, offering concrete achievements you have earned is advantageous. Leadership abilities and teamwork experiences are important to some schools so they may ask you about your activities in those areas as well.

To help you navigate this vast category of questions, we've categorized them into questions about being a doctor, being a team player, and being unique. This is perhaps the biggest category of questions so you will need to think and plan your responses accordingly. It is also important that you don't repeat information given in your primary application's essay and activity list as you answer these questions.

Being a Doctor

To prepare for these AU types of questions, you might identify three or four key influences or situations in your life that represent yourself. You might start with your childhood and then move into your college life in a chronological structure, or you might choose the most influential factors in an importance structure. You should definitely be prepared to discuss your interest in medicine above all other topics.

Questions to Ask Yourself about Being a Doctor

✓ What was a situation in which I first realized my dream of being a doctor?

✓ What specific experiences have I had to motivate my pursuit of medicine?

✓ What do I anticipate my role to be in the medical community as a doctor?

✓ What am I willing to do to achieve the goal of becoming a doctor?

✓ What have I already done to prepare myself for becoming a doctor?

✓ How have with others' sickness influenced me?

✓ How did that dream become a goal in my life? What have I done to achieve it?

✓ How do I view medicine? As research? As healing? As helping the unfortunate?

Develop several strong, well-written paragraphs. It is doubtful you will use these paragraphs in their entirety; instead, you are creating paragraphs that may be modified into specific secondary questions asking about your influences or background or motivations. The more questions you prepare for and answer concisely now with excellent examples, the easier your secondary applications will be since you will have the foundation for countless additional questions.

Being a Team Player

In medicine, doctors working together productively on a team can be advantageous for patients' health. In addition to your fellow doctors, you will have to effectively communicate with nurses and other support staff while meeting the requirements of the insurance companies and hospital administration. No successful doctor is an island of excellence in today's medical field. Hence, you must be an active collaborator in the pursuit of overall health. Because of this, working well with others on a team is a vital skill for a physician, and you should be able to demonstrate your ability in this area. In-class or out-of-class, what kind of group activities have you participated in? If you have leadership experience in such situations, it is even better! However, most importantly you must demonstrate your ability to be a team player successfully aiding a group in meeting a mutual goal. You should be able to explain the purpose of the group work and the function of your role.

Questions to Ask Yourself about Being a Team Player

✓ What have I learned about the importance of teamwork?

✓ What experiences have I had in being part of a team?

✓ What was my role on the team? How did I fulfill it?

✓ What did I do well in my and teamwork experiences? What did I need to learn?

✓ How have I demonstrated the capacity to work effectively with others?

✓ How have I demonstrated leadership ability?

✓ How can I apply these lessons to my medical school activities?

✓ How can I apply these lessons to my future as a physician?

Develop several strong examples of your teamwork activities. We suggest using those most related to medicine if you have them; if you don't, make sure to apply all the lessons you have learned to medical school or your future practice.

Being Unique

You are unique in your own way, so you will fit well with some schools, but not with others. Medical schools are concerned with both your success and with their own prosperity as well. They need to choose candidates who are able to excel academically plus fit into their particular environment.

Getting into a medical school requires more than just good grades and scores – you need to be a good fit. Therefore, the schools truly do want to understand you. To stand out from the others applying for the same few spots in these schools, it is important that you be both honest and original here. Your success requires you that you not only get into medical school but more importantly that you get into the right medical school for you.

Questions to Ask Yourself about Being Unique

- ✓ What unique attributes do I have?

- ✓ What is a rewarding experience I have had? Why was it rewarding?

- ✓ What volunteer experiences have I had which made a difference in the world?

- ✓ What significant academic achievements have I accomplished?

- ✓ What kind of research have I done?

- ✓ What non-academic achievements have I accomplished?

- ✓ How do I inspire others?

- ✓ How do I have fun?

It will be beneficial to demonstrate your unique characteristics to the schools that request secondary applications. You don't want to waste their time or your own. Don't worry about the characteristics or experiences that you do not have; instead, focus on who you are, what you have accomplished, and why you would be a fit for their schools.

Diversity Experiences – DE

Throughout the world, and especially in the current American landscape, working well with a diverse population is paramount to being successful in most professions; it is of particular importance in the medical field. In medical school, you will have to work well with peers from many socioeconomic environments, you will have to work well with professors from various specialties, and ultimately, you will be treating a diverse patient population throughout your career. You should be prepared to show multiple situations in which you have clearly communicated with a diverse population. You should be able to articulate some kind of experience with a diverse population whether such occurred in-class or out-of-class.

Be prepared to explain not only how diversity has affected your past, but also how it may affect your future as a doctor. Be as accurate as possible in your examples. If you are asked how you can contribute to a particular school, you will have to research the conditions of that school so that you can appropriately indicate how you can positively add to it. Remember, medical schools want candidates who will bring honor to the school as well as earn a degree.

Questions to Ask Yourself about Diversity Experiences

✓ Why is diversity important?

✓ What linguistic, social, educational, or cultural diversity have I experienced?

✓ How did the experience impact my life?

✓ How did this experience make me a better person? Student? Future physician?

✓ How will it aid my future ability in medical school or as a doctor?

✓ How will my previous experiences add to the diversity of the school that I attend?

Postbac Activities – PA

Many students have a time gap, often called the gap-year, between graduation and entering medical school. The MCAT is a seriously difficult test, and many students take a year just to prepare for it. Likewise, some students pursue other interests before applying to medical school. Such time lapses are a normal part of the process; nonetheless, any time gaps must be explained. If you have been out of school for a time, you will have to account for your time off. Also, you will need to elucidate what you have been doing to prepare yourself for the arduous task of becoming a physician and explain why you will still have an excellent level of scholarship ability when you return.

During this gap year, it is an excellent time to volunteer for activities. While getting your B.A., you might have been too busy studying the content to think about outside activities. If you don't have any, now would be the time to do something medically related.

Included in this category are required explanations if you are reapplying to medical schools after having not been accepted in the previous cycle. It is quite common for students to need to apply multiple times before getting in. If this is your case, make sure you are prepared to explain how you have been making yourself a more desirable candidate since the last application cycle.

> ### Questions to Ask Yourself about Postbac Activities
>
> ✓ Why have I been out of school for the length of time I have?
>
> ✓ What have I accomplished during this time?
>
> ✓ What specific things have I done to familiarize myself with the medical field?
>
> ✓ What volunteer activities have I participated in? How do these relate to medicine?
>
> ✓ How has this time out of school contributed to my overall development?
>
> ✓ How will this time positively affect my ability in medical school?
>
> ✓ If I am reapplying, why am I more qualified in this application than previously?

Challenging Situations – CS

Everyone has weaknesses of one kind or another. The key to a successful presentation is not to try to hide any weakness, but to acknowledge it boldly, and then explain why this weakness can, in fact, be a strength. In doing so, consider what have you learned from your weakness. Have you overcome it? If not entirely, what part of it have you mastered? How can this weakness actually show that you are stronger for experiencing it? This is a significant category, and you can expect at least one secondary question from it. It's important to pick valid weaknesses carefully as this is the category in which many applicants respond poorly.

> ### Questions to Ask Yourself about Challenging Situations
>
> ✓ About Failure - How have I dealt with criticism? How have I dealt with failure? How has that made me a better person? How will it make me a better physician?
>
> ✓ About Low Course Grade, GPA or MCAT - What were the circumstances? What did I learn? How will this enable me to succeed in medical school?
>
> ✓ About Time Off School - What were the circumstances? What did I learn? How will this enable me to succeed in medical school?
>
> ✓ About Reapplication - Why am I a stronger candidate now than I was before? How will this make me a better physician?

Future Plans - FP

Another common secondary question asks about where you see yourself in five, ten, or even fifteen years. This kind of question has multiple aspects to consider. The first is that you have to project your success. If you haven't thought beyond getting into medical school, then you might not make it through the grueling matriculation process. You have to see yourself at the end of the process, where you will be practicing, and what kind of practice you plan to have. Will you do pro-bono work or have yacht parties? Will you work in an urban ER or an exclusive plastic surgery office? Such dreams reveal what kind of person you are and what kind of doctor you may be. There is not really a right or wrong answer as there is every kind of doctor in the world. It is important that you be true to your own dreams since these are what will get you through the long, arduous days and nights of study. At five years, you should be almost finished with school, having picked your specialty and preparing to or having just started your residency. At ten years, you will be done with your schooling and will be beginning your practice. At fifteen years, you will have several years of experience as a medical practitioner.

Questions to Ask Yourself about Future Plans

✓ How will I manage the work-life balance?

✓ What kind of medicine do I think I will practice?

✓ What kind of work activities might I be involved in?

✓ What activities besides work do I see myself being involved in?

✓ What is a five-year goal or dream? Ten-year? Fifteen-year?

Keep in mind that your goals may change during your education, and that is ok. You are not locked into the plans and goals you mention now. Rather these ideas give insight into who you are, which may change a little outwardly, but probably will not change inwardly at the core of your personality.

School Specific – SS

Everyone likes to believe that he or she is special, the only one that matters. Medical schools are no different than the rest of us. While there may be one or two schools that you prefer, you probably would be happy getting accepted to any school that you applied to. Needless to say, that is never a good thing to tell a person, nor a school. Instead, you want the school to which you are sending your secondary application to feel like it is the best, most perfect fit for you and you for them. You will need to know details about specific programs for each school that you apply to in order to demonstrate why that school is your choice. As you consider this section, think about why you applied to each specific school. Review its mission statement. Look up the programs offered and find something that interests you. Look at the student body demographics. What can you add to that?

Questions to Ask Yourself about School Specifics

✓ How does this school's mission statement or philosophy directly impact me?

✓ How might I add to the student body diversity there?

✓ How can this school help me achieve my dream? Do I want to stay in that state?

✓ What program here interests me? How could I add to that program?

This is a category that you might want to wait to prepare for until you actually have the secondary application requested by the school. It will take you a lot of time to research each school, and there is now guarantee that every school you apply to will request your secondary application. Once you have received the secondary application, you can spend the appropriate amount of time researching that school. The more you can show you know about the school, the better choice you will be.

Other - O

The Other category is the most diverse, so perhaps the most difficult to prepare for in advance. Some topics in this category are financial information requests, family history, criminal history, grade discrepancies, and interview availability. Also, in this category are those schools whose previously given secondary questions were not readily available and so are unknown. Most importantly is a section to add anything you would wish the committee to know. If you have a particular weakness, for example, a low score on one section of the MCAT, a low score in a science class, or a re-application for medical school, this would be the place to explain it. For this category, if you have some extenuating circumstance that you need to explain, then absolutely take the time to write it well. Otherwise, most of the Other category questions will be more efficiently prepared once you receive them in the secondary application responses.

Review *Checklist 8: Secondary Application Preparation* in Chapter 9: Utilize Checklists to make sure you have sufficient answers developed.

Mrs. C's Tips: Answering Questions

From Mrs. C's experience, she has noticed that one of the most common reasons students don't do well on writing assignments or tests is they don't answer the question explicitly and comprehensively. It is easy to talk around a reply or give off-topic information. Make sure in your responses you're giving examples to respond to the particular question being asked. Moreover to give the most useful answer, make sure you provide specific details to make the example meaningful. For instance, when asked to explain his leadership ability, Lucas replied that he "led a group of students performing easy-to-do, at-home experiments so that the children attending the event could further their interest in chemistry. Because of that success, the group created the Chemistry Kicks Acid Youtube channel, posting child-friendly chemistry experiments." Hence, he provided detailed examples of the experiments with "easy to do" and "at home" adjectives. He also provides the name of the group's YouTube channel "Chemistry Kicks Acid." This example is relevant, interesting, believable, and specific thus actually illuminating his leadership ability. Whatever experience you are writing about, make sure that you stay on topic and give excellent examples!

Use the Categories

As you look through the secondary questions for the various schools that you have applied to, you'll find many repeated topics and similar issues. There may be a few unexpected outlier questions; however, if you focus on these 7 core categories, you should be able to create some solid responses that you can then modify as needed for individual schools.

Since you now have a general idea of the categories and have some questions to ask yourself regarding your own experience, let's look at more detailed examples of how to use this information in your preparation.

Review the excerpt below from *Chart 6: Secondary Application Questions*. Note to the school number and name in bold text at the top of the chart and the category indicated to the left of the question.

21	**George Washington University**
PB	3. For the application cycle, please indicate activities, academics, employment, or other occupations to account for full-time activity (approx. 30-40 hours per week).
AU	4. What is your most significant achievement outside the classroom?
CS DE	5. What makes you a unique individual? What challenges have you faced? How will these factors help you contribute to the diversity of the student body at GW?

The following are Lucas' answers to these 3 questions with the category indicate on the left:

PB	I will keep volunteering at UC Irvine Medical Center and my rotation in the acute surgical care unit. Simultaneously, in my interning job at Joshua Medical Group, I will continue the weekly senior activities. Plus, I will help to organize the clinic's Senior Health Fair as well as begin working as a medical scribe. Beside my medical-related work, I will remain working at OCC, tutoring multiple subjects. Moreover, I will also TA for general chemistry classes during this time, so that I can review old materials and stay sharp at my job as a tutor. In my free time, I enjoy working to improve the Chemplate Company and would like to partner with more colleges, corporations, and companies to further introduce Chemplate to more students in need.
AU	At UC Berkeley, I combined my passion for inventing things with my chemistry knowledge and entrepreneurship to invent the Chemplate, a plastic template for drawing organic molecules, and founded Chemplate Company. Along this unique journey, I acquired many useful skills in international communication, marketing, and multitasking. Moreover, it was the ups and downs of the business that taught me the most valuable lesson, which impacted my life strongly: I learned that failure is not only an integral part of success but also an important one. This reminds me that I need to be more careful in every step I take, to appreciate what I have already had, and last but not least, to embrace failure and keep moving on to achieve my final goal.
CS DE	I am bilingual, but more accurately, I am bicultural; every day I juggle between two identities. At school, I am Lucas; I speak English and hang out with friends who moved out of their house and became independent when they turned 18. At home, I am Thuan and speak Vietnamese to my parents. As the many differences in the two value systems clash frequently, I have to reconcile them every day, from small errands such as choosing the food to eat with my parents at the mall to big decisions such as how I am going to take care of my parents when they age. With practice, I have managed to harmonize these conflicts while still honoring my original culture. **Being bicultural has taught me the skills to** resolve cultural conflicts, and I believe if I can handle these two identities at once, I can blend smoothly from one cultural group to another in medical school, to overcome possible interpersonal difficulties arising in a team setting, and to help my peers to successfully communicate with each other as well as with the faculty.

Lucas was able to modify those answers as needed to make them fit the new incoming secondaries. This modification can be seen in his secondary answer to a question from the Brown excerpt from *the Chart 6: Secondary Application Questions*.

5	**Brown (Warren Alpert)**
PB	1. Summarize your activities for the academic year and describe how they are preparing you for a medical career
DE	2. How will your unique attributes add to the overall diversity of the Alpert Medical School community?

While this PB question for Brown is similar to the previous George Washington PB question, Lucas' answer is modified slightly to respond to exactly what Brown is requesting; the similarities have been bolded in the Brown response below. Because the core information for both questions is the same, Lucas saved time and effort, yet still created an original response for this particular secondary question.

PB

In the 2014-2015 academic year, **I will continue working at Orange Coast College's Student Success Center tutoring chemistry, biology, and physics and volunteering as a TA for general and organic chemistry labs.** Remaining in an academic environment will enable me to repeatedly refresh my core science knowledge while disseminating this information as a tutor to undergraduates will help me better communicate with my peers in medical school. Moreover, **I will also continue my medical volunteering at the UC Irvine Medical Center.** As a dispatcher, I will develop my ability to multitask in a fast-paced environment with a diverse population. Also, as I rotate in the acute care unit of the hospital, I will develop my tolerance for difficult situations helping patients in severe pain. **Simultaneously, as an intern at the Joshua Medical Group**, I will be shadowing Dr. Wong in his private practice and interpreting for him in the Vietnamese community in Buena Park. These activities will enrich my medical knowledge about diseases and treatments, especially diabetes, as well as demonstrate communication skills between a practicing physician and patients. Additionally, working as Dr. Wong's medical scribe and assistant, I will be able to take an active part in some of the daily operations of the clinic, offering me complementary opportunities to prepare for medical school. Besides these medical-related activities, **I will further develop Chemplate Company**. In this endeavor, I will continue to strengthen my time management skills, communication capability, and presentation proficiency. These skills will greatly enhance my personal characteristics so that I can adapt rapidly and perform excellently in medical school.

In this DE response for Brown, which allowed 2000 characters with spaces, Lucas combined the George Washington responses from the AU and CS/DE categories. With slight modifications, these polished paragraphs were able to be applied in multiple situations as demonstrated below in the Brown secondary response.

DE

> I am bilingual, but more accurately, I am bicultural; every day I juggle between two identities. At school, I am Lucas; I speak English and hang out with friends who moved out of their house and became independent when they turned 18. At home, I am Thuan and speak Vietnamese to my parents, who expect me to take care of them when they age. As the many differences in the two value systems clash frequently, I have to reconcile them every day. With constant practice, I have managed to harmonize this dissonance, thriving as an American student while still honoring my original culture. **Being bicultural has taught me the skills to** resolve cultural conflicts, and I believe if I can handle these two identities at once, I can blend smoothly from one cultural group to another in medical school, to overcome possible interpersonal difficulties arising in a team setting, and to help my peers to successfully communicate with each other as well as with the faculty at Alpert Medical School.
>
> Furthermore, inventing the Chemplate and managing my own business have been the most daring but most beneficial decisions I have ever made. Through this exciting **entrepreneurial** journey, the Chemplate Company has trained me with so many valuable life skills and taught me multiple lessons that ultimately have given me wisdom. Last but not least, Template let me experience multiple failures in my entrepreneurship to teach me the significant lesson that failure is part of life. I have learned not to be discouraged when I could not make an impression with my customers, but always give my all to everything I do so that I would not regret anything later. It is not a reach to say that Chemplate has given me a positive look on life and the drive to follow through with my goal, which will enhance my personality to benefit the diverse student population **at Alpert Medical School.**

Assuredly, not all questions can be prepared for in advance; there will be some specific questions you will have to compose at the time the secondary comes in. Some medical schools may ask about specific medical scenarios or unexpected philosophical queries. Nevertheless, a large part of your secondary responses can be planned for so that you have time to develop excellent answers. It is vital to be organized regardless so that once the interviews start coming in, you can review what you said and be prepared to elaborate as needed and perhaps cover missing aspects of your application package that were not previously stressed.

Have Effective Organization

The correlation between being organized and submitting successful secondaries cannot be emphasized enough. It is vital to your success that you effectively organize your information so that you can get your secondary application out on time and without error.

To stay organized in his application cycle, before he received a single secondary application, Lucas wrote four to five general paragraphs for each of the given seven categories and filed them under type AU.doc or CS.doc. Then when the secondary response questions came in, these pre-prepared responses were organized and ready to be modified or edited as needed.

Once you start receiving the secondary applications, you may see repeated topics in the questions. To efficiently organize all your available information, as you write each response, save it under the school's name. Then, as new secondary questions come in, you can check to see if you have already answered such a question. For example Duke (#13), Stony Brook (#61), the University of Washington (#130) and Wake Forest (#135) all ask very similar questions requesting you to describe an obstacle you overcame. If you stay organized and have the answer the Duke question readily accessible and then weeks later, you must answer the University of Washington secondary question, your work is partially completed before you even start that question.

Of course, you have to be able to easily find the original response! So having a filing system for your pre-written paragraphs will enable you to adapt them to each secondary question. This is why taking time in the beginning to be organized and then taking time as you go to stay organized can save you time, effort, and energy as the process goes on. If you have applied to thirty to forty medical schools, the incoming secondary responses can be overwhelming after a while. Nonetheless, if you follow our suggestions, the process will be more easily managed and will be quite beneficial to you in the long run as you prepare for your interviews.

The Chapter 10: Utilize Charts *Chart 1 Application & Interview Tracking* will help you organize your secondary applications and interviews. You can use this form or create your own if you find it more helpful. What matters isn't the exact method you use, but rather that you find some way to be organized! To stay organized, enter the information for each school and the date as each one comes in, and write the due date next to it. Give yourself a turnover deadline and stick with it. Also, jot down any username and password that you create for that secondary, so you don't forget the information the next time you log in. After you finish the secondary, mark the submitted box with the date, and update the interview box regularly. If you get an interview from the school, check the box. Cross out the school to eliminate it from the list if you don't get in.

We suggest you submit each secondary response within three days minimum to a week maximum. You will probably be submitting for weeks. Once all of your secondary applications are sent, you must wait for the interview requests.

Mrs. C's Tips: Indispensable Organization

By this point in your academic career, you too have learned the importance of organization and even if you're not great at it, you have had enough organizational skill to succeed in your undergraduate years, or you wouldn't be applying to medical school. Now is the time to demonstrate all the techniques and strategies you have mastered to this point! This application process is just the beginning of your medical journey. Keeping up with all the academic courses, physical demands, and emotional stresses in medical school will require expert organizational skills. The more you can be organized with your materials, your time, and your efforts, the better off you'll be. Don't think about just getting through this application process; instead, look at this as a primer for the organization needed in school!

CHAPTER 5: PREPARE FOR INTERVIEWS
September - December

If you have followed our recommendations for school selection, then you should plan on getting school interviews and must prepare in advance for them. For the previous sections of your application, all your responses were planned in advance and written carefully whereas your interviews will be more spontaneous. Despite the nature of the interview process, you can still prepare to be evaluated on how you look, how you speak, and how well you respond to unexpected questions. Unless you have a lot of practice with public speaking, the interview process may very well be the most stressful aspect. Luckily, there are things you can do to prepare yourself and decrease your stress. This chapter provides various techniques through three steps for you to be the most prepared you can for your school interviews.

Step 1: Plan

<u>First Plan Your Words</u>

While each school will have their own particularities and preferences for medical school candidates, all schools will want some basic traits. If you have made it through the secondary process, then you have what it takes to be a doctor. But the question remains, do you have what it takes to fully and successfully participate in a specific school's program? All schools seek to answer these four questions when interviewing potential students:

Schools' Questions

1. How will you fit in their program?
2. How will you achieve success in their program?
3. How can you support and promote their program?
4. How will you bring honor and prestige to their program?

Therefore, it is essential that you keep these four questions in mind at all times as you formulate your answers to sample questions and in the actual interview. Even more than the secondary responses, for interviews, you need to research all available information on that school and be prepared to demonstrate why you are the perfect fit for that school at this time.

In addition to school-specific questions, there are many generalized questions that you can prepare for, much like you did for the secondary responses. Based on our own research and Lucas' actual interviews, we have organized ninety-five general interview questions into five categories to help you organize your information and maximize your preparation. The largest category of Personal Characteristics is comprised of forty-five questions divided into the subcategories of Personal Background, Individual Characteristics, Thought Processes, Acquired Activities, and Overcoming Adversity. The next largest category of Healthcare Issues is comprised of twenty questions divided into the subcategories of You, Community, and World. The last three categories Medical Scenarios, School Specifics, and Your Questions are comprised of ten questions each. Each of these five categories covers important aspects of your suitability for medical school. See Chapter 10: Utilize Charts, *Chart 7: Practice Interview Questions.*

Much of the information in Category 1: Personal Characteristics and Category 4: School Specifics you have probably already covered in your secondary application preparation. Now you are just condensing it and sorting out the most compelling examples of your points. You may have even covered some of Category 2: Healthcare Issues as well. However, Category 3: Medical Scenarios and Category 5: Your Questions may be new to you.

We suggest you prepare a response for each of the ninety-five questions and practice succinctly answering them. Lucas used notecards and carried them around to practice in preparation for his interviews. Many study apps are also available. At this point, you know how you study best. The key is to have adequate responses prepared.

To do that, you must ascertain not just what information is being requested from you, but also, in which context you will be giving your answer. Every question you answer has a deeper subtext embedded in the answer. To give good answers, you also must identify possible deeper meanings that you give in your response. Analyzing one's own answers can be a difficult thing to do.

Consider the basic question: discuss a book that you have read lately and explain why. Obviously, you need to pick a book and explain why you've read it. Simple, right? However, even this self-explanatory question reveals so much more than just your book choice. Let's look at the process together to further your understanding.

Consider the complete question from Category 1: Personal Characteristics, Subcategory: Thought Processes Question #6: "What book have you read for pleasure lately. Why did you select it? Did you like it? Explain."

Lucas' Response: The most recent book that I read was *The Hunger Games* by Suzanne Collins. The book is about a teenage girl, Katniss Everdeen, born into a slave zone under the dictatorship of the Capitol people, and through a revolution with a strong and determined mind has achieved freedom. I picked the book because I was born in Viet Nam, a developing country and have witnessed other teenagers suffering like the characters in the story. Thus, I sympathized and felt a strong connection with the characters. More importantly, the book taught me a very valuable lesson that with a determined mind and hard work, victory is achievable.

Lucas answered the question concretely by supplying a specific popular fictional novel he read over the summer. He also gives reasons for choosing this book and what he learned from it. On the surface, he literally answered answer the question. Additionally, if we look more analytically into this answer, we can glean other insight into who he is now and who he will be as a future doctor.

Lucas' Response Reveals

✓ He is influenced by popular culture, which demonstrates his interests outside medicine.

✓ He is not gender-biased because the heroine is female, which demonstrates his diversity competence.

✓ He values freedom, determination, and hard work, which will help him in medical school.

✓ He can personalize and apply information to his own background and future situations, which demonstrates critical thinking capability.

✓ He is willing to think about difficult issues like combat and death, which will be relevant as a physician.

How might you answer this question?

Your Response Will Reveal

✓ What interests you outside of academia, which reveals how balanced you are in life and how current you are with culture.

✓ How prepared you are for non-medical questions, which reveals your work ethic, preparation abilities, and balance in life.

✓ How your mind works and what engages you, which reveals how you think now and may think as a future doctor.

✓ Whether you can learn life lessons outside of the classroom, which reveals your drive for self-improvement and critical thinking.

✓ Whether you can personalize and apply general information to your life, which reveals critical thinking ability.

✓ Whether you are intrinsically motivated to self-improve or only do things when assigned in class, which reveals your drive for excellence and study habits.

All of these insights into you can be revealed from just one book choice! From this example, you can see that every question has multiple layers that need to be considered. This is why you must prepare in advance. If you just answer off the top of your head in an interview situation, who knows what subtext you may give!

The interview is such a valuable tool for acceptance into medical school. Given this information, think about your answers not only regarding the obvious explicit responses and but also the deeper implicit meanings you might disclose with your reply.

In addition to preparing answers to the sample questions we have provided in *Chart 7: Practice Interview Questions* in Chapter 10: Utilize Charts, you should practice re-wording the questions in various ways to get a sense of how the same information might be differently requested. Pick out the key concept of the question, and consider other ways it could be asked.

For example, consider Category 1: Personal Characteristics, Subcategory: Overcoming Adversity Question # 5, "Explain a failure and what you learned." The key concepts here are what constitutes failure for you and how you handle it.

One question may be asked in various ways, but the answers can be the same. To help you prepare, think about the underlining information being asked. If you understand what is being asked of you, then you can give the relevant information with appropriate context.

Multiple Ways to Ask the Same Question

✓ Discuss a time you struggled to succeed. What happened?

✓ Give an example of a failed endeavor. How did you move on?

✓ What kind of defeat have you encountered? Explain.

✓ How have you failed in your life? How did you overcome it?

Although each one was worded rather differently, Lucas was asked a question about failure in each one of his interviews. For this kind of question, you want to show that you can overcome failure in a productive and progressive manner as he did in his response. Some form of this question will probably be asked in your interviews as well.

How might you answer this question?

Let's consider some other practical examples. Each of the following examples includes Lucas' response, Mrs. C's analysis of that response, and your possible application of the question. Keep in mind that these examples are in no way supposed to be considered the perfect examples. As always, examples are just that – examples. It's imperative that you apply the information to your life and your experiences.

Example # 1

Category 1: Personal Characteristics, Subcategory: Individual Characteristic, Q # 1 – Question: Who are you? If you were an animal, what type would you be?

Lucas' Response: If I were an animal, I would be an okapi. I am bicultural; every day I juggle between two identities, and instead of choosing between the two, integrating them is the right thing to do, so I try to accommodate the American while maintaining authenticity in the Vietnamese. At school, I am Lucas; I speak English and hang out with friends who moved out of their homes and became independent when they turned 18. In contrast, at home, I am Thuan and speak Vietnamese to my parents, who expect me to take care of them when they age. With constant practice, I have managed to harmonize this dissonance between the two value systems, thriving as an American student while still honoring my original culture. Thus, these experiences have caused me to identify with the African "Okapi," a unique fusion of animals in nature with a horse-like body, striped zebra-like legs, and a longish neck with the head of a giraffe; like the Okapi I am a blend of many parts, which make me unique and interesting.

This answer incorporated information that Lucas had prepared for his secondary applications. He had previously responded to the challenge of being bi-cultural and bi-lingual. To best respond to this interview question, he looked for an animal that could represent his duality and discovered the African okapi, an animal that looks like a cross between a giraffe, zebra, and horse. This answer shows his thoughtfulness and depth which is important as he takes very little in life lightly. Thus, with this one answer, the interviewers can see that he is a deep thinker, who is loyal to both his cultural influences.

However you answer this question, you want it to reflect who you are and how you think. Not only the words themselves, but even the choice of animal reveals details about your nature. There is really no right or wrong answer; instead, the response shows what kind of person you are, thus showing what kind of doctor you will become. There is every kind of doctor, so be true to yourself.

How might you answer this question?

Example # 2

Category 1: Personal Characteristics, Subcategory: Thought Processes, Q # 5 – Question: Who has been the most influential person in the last 100 years? Why?

Lucas' Response: I would say Steve Jobs because I can relate to him in many ways. First, he is a self-made man who built a company that changes the world from his empty hands. Also, he was determined to pursue his dream and worked his absolutely best to achieve his dream. Last but not least, I admired his great vision as well as his daring move to create and follow his own path, leaving behind the traditional route of education that does not fit him, because isolating yourself from the norm is a very difficult thing to do

While Lucas is very driven to pursue a career in medicine, he is not limited to only that interest. Hence, he chose someone outside of medicine who influenced him and explained why. Lucas too is a self-made man going against the norm of an immigrant ESL student to rise up and become an American doctor practicing in English rather than his native language. He too has demonstrated excellence in pursuit of this dream. He too has a vision and dares to follow his own path, but instead of technology, his path will be medicine. Even though many find Jobs inspirational, Lucas still personalizes the impact by applying it directly to himself rather than the world in general. This is a daring move to pick someone so famous and so outside of medicine. Nevertheless, this is the person whom Lucas sincerely believed provided the most inspiration for him personally, so Steve Jobs was his selection.

However you answer this question, you should have an honest response. It should be someone that you can relate to, and you should personalize the response as much as possible. Remember, everything you choose reveals things about yourself. Lucas was even wearing his Apple Watch during the interview further subtlety demonstrating Job's influence. Consistency and genuineness should be keys to your own answers too.

How might you answer this question?

Example # 3

Category 1: Personal Characteristics, Subcategory: Acquired Activities, Q # 1 – Question: Explain a situation when you were working in a diverse environment. What did you learn?

Lucas' Response: When I began my internship at Joshua Medical Group, the very first task given to us was to organize the clinic's Senior Health Fair to promote a healthy lifestyle within the senior community. Since most of the interns were freshmen in college, and I had already graduated, working with them was an interesting experience. The ways that they operated were more tech savvy, so I had to start using new social media to quickly adapt to their methods. In addition, I was in charge of the entertainment, coordinating four high school volunteers to operate at four different game booths. Surprisingly, virtually all of the seniors participating in this event spoke either only Mandarin or Cantonese and very little English, but none of us speaks any Chinese. Nonetheless, by smiling in combination with multiple gestures to communicate and a positive attitude, the seniors felt very welcomed and took part in the game very enthusiastically, leading to a very successful event. Through this experience, I became more spontaneous, adapting and shifting quickly between unpredictable situations. I also learned that with an optimistic attitude toward difficulty, problems become easier to solve.

For this question, Lucas combined his relevant medical experience with teamwork to get the most out of his answer. He covered a broad range of diverse groups, using both age and language. He also showed his leadership ability through the experience given. Perhaps most importantly, the positive lesson he learned can directly apply to the medical profession since doctors must adapt quickly to changing situations. This answer highlights many important aspects of Lucas' strengths, including teamwork, leadership, adaptability, and a positive attitude.

However you choose to answer such a question, try to highlight strengths in your own situation as well as tie it, if possible, to medical school. The more you can integrate your responses, the better they will be. Remember, every single question, regardless of the content, should show why you out of all applicants are a good fit for that institution.

How might you answer this question?

Example # 4

Category 1: Personal Characteristics, Subcategory: Overcoming Adversity, Q # 5 – Question: Explain a situation when you experienced failure. What did you learn?

Lucas' Response: As a human being constantly trying to improve, I have experienced quite a lot of failure through the process. At first, it was very frustrating. However, realizing that being sad over failure would not help me improve at all, I tried to rationalize the situations to learn from them. Also, I always try my best at everything that I do, so that later on I won't look back and regret that I didn't give it my best. For example, when I received my MCAT verbal reasoning score, I was very frustrated with the low result. However, I did try the absolute best that I could. Thus, I got over the frustration and mapped out a plan to do more reading to improve my reading speed as well as comprehension

Here Lucas made a tactical decision. Because his MCAT verbal reasoning score was less than average, he knew it would be an issue in getting accepted to medical school. Thus, whenever possible, he took the opportunity to show that that particular weakness didn't mean he was a weak candidate. He used that as a very real example of a failure. With this response, he demonstrated that failure would not paralyze him nor defeat him but that he would acknowledge it, learn from it, and prosper despite it. It can be scary to discuss a real failure, but doing so demonstrates a strong will to succeed.

However you answer this kind of question, make sure that you have chosen a good example of failure, something that you truly learned from and that affected your life in a meaningful way. Everyone fails; it is the response to the failure that reveals who a person is, not the failure itself. If you have a glaring weakness in your application packet, this would be a good time to bring it out. Don't ignore the elephant in the room, but bring attention to it instead!

How might you answer this question?

Example # 5

Category 2: Healthcare Issues, Subcategory: You, Q # 13 – Question: How could you affect the healthcare system?

Lucas' Response: As a physician, I am a small cell in the multicellular healthcare organism. Thus, I think the best way to affect the healthcare system is to try my best to fulfill my responsibility first and then continue in constantly learning and exploring new things to drive the system forward.

With this response, Lucas demonstrates his focus on biology and chemistry, which is his strong science background. He also demonstrates his analytic rather than emotional response to medicine. While he does want to help people, he isn't only emotionally driven to do so, and his answer reveals this about him. He knows even before he begins medical school that it is doubtful that he will be a family physician, but may be a surgeon or perhaps even researcher, a more distant medical role. His response also shows a commitment to excellence in his treatment of patients and in his continued education. Both of these are excellent characteristics.

However you answer this question, the response should be consistent with who you are, what you believe, and what your goals are. There is really no right or wrong answer; the answer reveals the kind of doctor you will be. It takes all kinds, so be true to your goals.

How might you answer this question?

Example # 6

Category 3: Medical Scenarios, Q # 3 – Question: If there were an accident on the road, would you stop and help the victims, knowing that you doing so might lead to a malpractice claim against you?

Lucas' Response: As a human being, I think everybody has a tendency to stop and give out a hand when help is needed. I am no exception. If I happened to get stuck in traffic due to a car accident and the emergency team could not get there yet, I would help get the victims into a stable condition so that the EMT team could help them faster when they get there. Even though there is a risk that I might get sued, I would still help that victim while being extra careful so that there is little chance that the victims later can file a malpractice claim

Given Lucas' tendency to analytic responses, it is important to also show the compassionate side of his personality, so in this answer, he says he would stop and help. It is important to present a well-balanced picture of yourself, and he does this here. Nonetheless, he still acknowledges the legality of possibly being sued; since he is a pragmatic man, he would have thought of that. In helping the stranger despite the fear of malpractice, he demonstrates the importance of aiding those in need, yet limits his contribution to what is required by saying he would turn the patient over to the appropriate medical team when they arrive. Thus, once again he shows who he would be as a doctor through what he values.

However you answer the question, the response will reveal what you value, and thus what kind of student and doctor you will be. It is important not to search for an answer you think the committee desires. You must be true to yourself and represent your values. These kinds of ethical dilemmas are faced by doctors every day, so you must figure out what it is you believe. Always keep in mind that the school is ultimately trying to find the best fit for their mission and program.

How might you answer this question?

Lucas' example responses are not meant to be used as the correct way to answer any questions. There is very little right or wrong in this process. If your answers are drastically different from his, then you are on an appropriate track! Now more than ever you must be authentic and honest. Remember, perhaps the most important thing in the interview process is to be genuine. You will have no certainty regarding what applicant the school is looking for. You must be who you are and express what you believe. Succeeding in medical school will probably be the hardest thing you ever do. You don't want to add to that stress a situation in which you are trying to be something you aren't. There is every kind of doctor out there; there is room in the profession for whatever kind of doctor you wish to be.

What kind of doctor do you want to be?

If you don't fit in at one school, you don't want to go there. Statistically, it is near impossible to transfer from one medical school to another, and even rarer to drop out and then go back to medical school. It is imperative, not just for the school's success, but also for your own success that the match between the school and student be a good one. Trying to guess what a school is looking for is a recipe for failure. Instead, answer these practice questions honestly yet intelligently. If you are given an offer, you can confidently go forth knowing that this school would be a good one for you.

Next Plan Your Budget

Until this point, except for your initial application fees, there has been little need for money. Unfortunately, that has now changed. Interviewing, especially out-of-state, can be very expensive. This is an expense that you simply must accept as part of the process. How much you will need varies on a multitude of factors including location, number of interviews, and resources available. We can provide some general guidelines for things to consider, but the actual dollar amount will depend on your exact situation. Here are the categories you need to plan for.

Your Look

Maybe you already have appropriate clothing in your closet, but maybe you don't. Most undergraduate students are not going to class in business wear, and your jeans and tee-shirt will not be appropriate here. While you don't have to look like a magazine cover model, you do want to present a professional, attractive image. You can invest a chunk of money and outfit yourself with a new look. You can mix expensive and inexpensive pieces. You can buy used or borrow from friends. There are many options available for you now. This should be a one-time purchase that meets several interview requirements. Plan to acquire the best clothing and accessories that your budget will allow.

Your Transportation

If you do attend out-of-state interviews, costs can add up quickly. All of Lucas' seven interviews were out-of-state, so there was a lot of flying involved. If the school you are attending is in a small town, it could save you money to fly to a larger hub airport and drive to the smaller town rather than flying directly into the smaller airport. Don't forget the baggage check fees! In addition to plane fare, you will probably need to rent a car when you arrive. You'll need money for gas and perhaps toll roads as well. While it would be nice to have multiple interviews in the same out-of-state location at the same time, if you got interviews at UCLA and UCI in the same week, for instance, this might not be possible. While some schools do ask for schedule considerations, others don't. You might be interviewing at UCLA in December and UCI in February, thus needing two California trips. Therefore, budget your funds for travel accordingly.

Your Lodging

If you are going out-of-state, you will most likely be staying a day or two. Some schools may offer help with your accommodations; at one of Lucas' interviews, he was able to stay with a medical student on campus, thus saving money and learning about the school at the same time. If you are unfamiliar with the area, you might not know where to stay, so use the Internet to help you. Yelp is a great resource for reviews. Staying in a college town may be more costly than staying in another nearby town. You have to weigh the cost of convenience against the actual dollar amount.

Your Food

Some schools may provide breakfast or lunch for you. Regardless, for the most part, you are own your own. If you are on a tight budget, you can take snacks with you to save money. Energy bars, dried fruit, and packaged nuts can be packed in carry-on or checked luggage and substantially cut down on costs. While not stylish, this is one area where you can definitely reduce spending. Do, however, make sure to eat! You don't want to bomb an interview because of brain fog due to hunger!

Your Time

If you are working, you will have to miss work. Don't expect to piggyback all your interviews in a tight time frame. Lucas' interviews occurred over a 5-month period. If you are on a tight monthly budget, missing that income could affect you, so plan accordingly.

Your Money

If you are going out-of-town, plan for some emergency funds. Tipping your housekeeping, taxi drivers, or restaurant servers could be required. You might have to pay for unexpected parking. Perhaps you will want to sight see as well. Wherever you go, you may want to buy a souvenir from the school. All these costs add up. Remember, these interview costs are an investment in your future. You can go hog wild or cheap, but you have to go!

Mrs. C's Tips: Travel Budgeting

The entire application process is a financial investment. On the one hand, flying all over the country to interview at different schools will be expensive. On the other hand, you want to make sure that get into the best possible school you can regardless of the cost. Lucas actually declined to attend an interview in New York. The invitation to interview came late in the cycle, and he had already traveled to seven schools. He weighed the cost of travel and being away from his job against the possibility of getting accepted into that school and then decided to forgo that interview because he'd already been accepted to three schools and waitlisted at another. Be aware that there is no guarantee that you will get accepted to every school where you interview. Being waitlisted is also a real possibility. Consider this as you plan your travel.

Then Plan Your Overall Look

Medical school is graduate school, which means that formal apparel will be required for the interview. You won't be wearing scrubs for a while yet! Presenting yourself professionally is a very real part of the interviewing process. It is generally accepted that the medical school interview is much like a high-powered job interview, which means you will need proper business attire. However, it is not necessary to spend thousands of dollars to be a fashion plate! Discount stores like Men's Warehouse and Nordstrom's Rack have name-brand looks for less. Even Wal-Mart and Target may have some appropriate clothing. If you don't mind used, consider Thrift Stores like Goodwill and Salvation Army. You may even already have things in your closet you can use. Put together the best outfit you have within your budget. Remember, right or wrong, you will be judged partly on your appearance, so plan carefully.

While specific characteristics may vary from school to school and region to region, some overall similarities can be planned for. Business attire rules for men and women follow similar guidelines, with some minor allowances for gender. If you have specific questions about your look, there is a plethora of information online about business wear that you can research. We did a Google search for "medical school interview wardrobe" and hundreds of images came up. The most important thing about your look is that you present yourself in a professional manner, and you are comfortable in your clothing.

After you have settled on your interview outfit, try it on. Wear it around the house. Have lunch in it. Take a picture of yourself in the outfit. Look at it objectively. Ask yourself do you look professional? Do I look like a doctor? Would you want yourself as a student? Here are some other practical considerations when thinking about what you should wear to an interview:

✓ Make sure you can walk in your shoes comfortably. There's nothing worse than having a bleeding blister as you walk into an interview.

✓ Make sure you can both stand and sit comfortably in your interview outfit. Your clothes shouldn't be too loose or too tight. Your collar should be comfortable. Your neckline should be appropriate. You don't want any embarrassing moments caused by your clothing in the middle of an interview.

✓ Make sure the details of your clothing are taken care of. Have no hanging threads or loose buttons. The hems of the pants should not drag on the floor. Details of your clothing do matter, so be attentive.

Our following Male Guidelines and Female Guidelines offer specific aspects of your look to consider depending on your gender.

Male Guidelines	
Head	You should have your hair trimmed. Facial hair should be trimmed and styled or removed completely
Top	You should plan to wear a suit jacket or sports coat. Choose neutral colors like blue, black, brown, or gray. Ties can be expressive with a pop of color but avoid garish prints. Avoid less formal button down collars. Dress shirts should be pressed and professional in a neutral color like white, cream, or light blue. A dress watch is permitted. Cufflinks are allowed, but not required.
Bottom	You should wear slacks that match your jacket. Pleated or not pleated pants are both allowed. You may wear a belt. Pants should be hemmed appropriately, not dragging on the ground.
Toes	You should match the color of the shoes to the belt. Black and brown are the most common choices. Formal dress shoes may or may not have laces and should be polished. Socks should match the color of the pants, usually black, brown, or navy. With gray pants, wear black socks if gray cannot be found.
Accessories	You should carry your cell phone in a bag or a phone clip, not the back pocket. Alternatively, it can be carried in the jacket pocket as well. A briefcase or classic leather backpack is allowed. Consider using a portfolio to carry any notes you may have. Nails should be neatly trimmed. A ring and watch are allowed. Use any cologne lightly. You may need a classic style dress coat for winter weather.

Female Guidelines	
Head	You should have your hair styled. If you have long hair, consider pulling it back into a chignon. Keep any hair accessories neutral, avoiding lots of bling. If your hair is colored, avoid trendy fashion choices. Earrings should be classically styled.
Top	You should wear a jacket. Consider neutral colors like blue, black, brown, or gray. Tops should be form fitted without revealing any cleavage. Consider adding color and personality to the top, but keep it simple. Any jewelry should be complementary yet understated.
Bottom	You should wear either a skirt or pants matching the top. For a skirt, the length should be at or below the knee. Pants should be hemmed appropriately, not dragging on the ground. Alternatively, a professional dress that matches the jacket is also allowed.
Toes	You should wear a closed toe and heel; a moderate heel is allowed. The shoe color should be a neutral one, matching the outfit. For all dark colors, black shoes are appropriate. For lighter colors, consider navy or gray. Bare legs are not considered professional attire, so wear appropriate matching neutral hose or trouser socks. A belt, if worn, should match the shoes.
Accessories	You should have a modest handbag that should complement the shoes. Consider using a classic portfolio to carry any notes you may have. Nails should be manicured and polished with classic colors. Avoid excessive jewelry in general; one ring per hand and a bracelet on one wrist are sufficient. Use any makeup and perfume lightly. You may need a classically styled dress coat for winter weather.

Mrs. C's Tips: Dressing the Part

Southern California is a relatively casual place where you'll find college instructors in blue jeans and students in class wearing shorts and sandals or even pajamas. Even so, there is nothing like a suit to make one feel professional and capable. When Mrs. C began her teaching career all those years ago, she invested a lot of money in two classic suits – one black and one brown. These outfits probably only get worn a couple of times a year, but they were well worth the financial outlay for her as a teaching professional. You may be hesitant to spend money on a suit you think you'll wear only for interviews. Actually though, as a medical school student, you may find many opportunities to wear this outfit. There will be your white coat ceremonies and award banquets. There will be internships interviews. You may even go on a formal date or two. And once you become a doctor, you will want to have a suit. Hence, get the best suit that you can afford and have it fitted appropriately. Buy the best accompanying accessories that you can afford as well. Good clothes never go out of style and will serve many functions in your upcoming career!

Finally Plan Your Travel

Perhaps you will only be interviewing in the state where you live, so this will be easy for you. However, it could be that you are traveling across the country to a place you've never been before. Perhaps like Lucas you're comfortable with travel and look upon it all as a big adventure or perhaps you're more like Mrs. C, one who much more prefers staying close to home. Either way, it's important that you are prepared for your trip. If you interview at more than one school, the costs can pile up pretty quickly too. Know that problems will occur! Plan for them!

The following are some areas we found useful in planning Lucas' out-of-state trips.

Transportation

If you are coming from out of town, you might not be familiar with the transportation choices in the area where you are visiting. In California for example, we don't consider distance the factor in getting to a place; instead, we consider the time of day and the traffic. Traveling fifteen miles could take as little time as forty-five minutes or as much time as two hours depending on the time of day and the traffic. In addition to possible time delays with traffic, the actual driving on crowded freeways can be very stressful if you're not used to such. Also, public transportation might be very different where you're going compared to where you're from. For example, in New York, you have to be comfortable with the subway, but in California, you might take an Uber car instead. Plan these details very carefully to save money and have the best experience you can. The more you can prepare in advance, the less stress you will experience the day of the interview.

> Questions to Ask Yourself about Transportation
> ✓ Do I have enough time in between flight connections?
> ✓ Do I have a backup plan in case my flight is delayed or my luggage gets lost?
> ✓ Does my insurance cover my rental car?

Lodging

This aspect of the trip may be expensive for you, depending on your travel distance. Some of the schools offer accommodations with a current student. If this is an available option, take it! You can really get a feel for the school by talking to actual students. Such information may help you make a choice between schools. If you are staying in a hotel, make sure your room will have an ironing board and iron. Most hotels do have such today, but it's nice to know for sure.

Also, make sure you know how to get from your hotel to the school. In some parts of the country, you'll be staying in a college town with the entire town revolving around the college; however, in places like Los Angeles, California, the college may be in a difficult to access area of the city. You should plan for traffic and weather. Lucas drove for over an hour in the Midwest through a slushy sleet storm on the way to one of his interviews. Having never driven in the snow previously, it certainly added some anxiety to his overall interview experience!

Questions to Ask Yourself about Lodging

✓ Does my lodging have all the amenities I need for my interview?

✓ Is my lodging in a secure area of town?

✓ Is my lodging reasonably close to my interview location?

✓ Is my lodging reasonably close to other areas I may want to visit?

Food

Don't wait until the last minute to think about sustenance! If you are like Lucas and can't have a coherent conversation without your morning Java, plan where you will get it. While many hotels now have coffee pots in the room, some don't. There might not be a Starbucks within walking distance to your room, or there might be one on every corner. Also, don't forget to think about eating. If you're like Mrs. C with her many dietary restrictions or like Lucas, who gets too nervous to eat before interviewing, you might have to bring your own snacks. Will your room have a refrigerator? Will you need one? Identify convenient restaurants in your area; don't assume your hotel will have room service or even a restaurant. Make sure you know where you can eat affordably.

Questions to Ask Yourself about Food

✓ Is there a convenient place near me for breakfast, lunch, and dinner?

✓ Is there a new place I want to try or my favorite comfort food available near me?

✓ Do I have snacks for the trip and my hotel room?

✓ Do I have throat lozenges or breath mints just in case?

Campus Activities

The schools are interviewing many applicants, so there will probably be activities available to you. There might be luncheons or conversations with current students. Lucas had the opportunity to attend a meet and greet with medical students for one of the schools where he interviewed. It was a great experience for him to ask current students questions about the school's program and lifestyle. Find out in advance if your school is offering such activities so you can allow enough time in your schedule to participate. Doing so will both demonstrate your interest in the school and ability to participate on a team as well as give you more vital information in case you are choosing between schools.

Even if the school doesn't offer any explicit get-togethers, you should plan to spend some time on the campus. If all works out well, you might have several schools to choose from and this time on the campus can really help you later to make a decision. You definitely want to go to the college bookstore and get a souvenir. Lucas brought Mrs. C a keychain from every school where he interviewed. You might want souvenirs too!

Questions to Ask Yourself about Campus Activities

✓ Is there an activity I can participate in?

✓ What do the students say about the program?

✓ What are the labs and classrooms on campus like?

✓ How easy is it to navigate on campus?

Weather

You will be interviewing in the winter months so you should take this into account in your travel plans. Winter storms don't care if you're trying to get to your interview. What will you do if your flight is delayed or canceled? One of Lucas' flights was delayed, and he arrived a day later than he had anticipated; luckily, we had planned for just such a problem so he simply missed a student-get-together but didn't miss the actual interview.

Furthermore, you should plan for cold weather for many American schools. Does the school area have cold weather? Do you have appropriate weather gear? Do you have a winter coat that complements your interview outfit? If you aren't used to winter weather, make sure you plan for it. Even with proper planning, however, situations can arise. Make sure you know who to contact in case there are problems with your travel. Plan ahead, but be flexible too!

```
┌─────────────────────────────────────────────────────────────┐
│           Questions to Ask Yourself about Weather            │
│   ✓ Do I have a backup plan for flight or trip delays?        │
│   ✓ Can I drive in winter conditions?                         │
│   ✓ Do I know who to contact if weather causes me to miss my  │
│     interview?                                                │
│   ✓ Do I have appropriate winter clothing?                    │
└─────────────────────────────────────────────────────────────┘
```

Technology

For us, our technology is a big part of lives, and we would be lost without our cell phones. Be aware that cell phone coverage in all regions of the country is not the same. You might want to check on your provider's coverage especially if you plan on using the Internet to help you get around with Google maps in an unfamiliar area. Because Mrs. C is directionally challenged and uses maps everywhere, even in her own town, so no internet would be a serious issue for her. Double check your phone coverage before you go! Also, make sure you have the means to keep your technology charged. Portable batteries are pretty inexpensive these days. Just make sure that you have what you need so that you don't have to panic and find an electronics store once you arrive.

Finally, remember your phone is more than a phone; it's also a representation of who you are and it presents an image to others. If you have some fun phone case like a Pikachu or Spiderman, you might want to remove it for the interview. It should also go without saying that you need to make sure that you can mute your phone so that it doesn't announce every Facebook post or other notice throughout your interview.

```
┌─────────────────────────────────────────────────────────────┐
│          Questions to Ask Yourself about Technology          │
│   ✓ Is my phone case appropriately styled to carry in an      │
│     interview?                                                │
│   ✓ Am I carrying a Wi-Fi hotspot just in case you don't      │
│     have access?                                              │
│   ✓ Does my cellular service have good coverage where I am    │
│     going?                                                    │
│   ✓ Do I have a portable charger or battery backup?           │
│   ✓ Do I know how to turn off my phone's sound?               │
└─────────────────────────────────────────────────────────────┘
```

There may be other aspects of your trip that we haven't mentioned. Since most of our information is based on our experience, we have a very distinctive point of view. As you go through the interview process if you encounter something we forgot, we'd love to hear it! Or if you're in Southern California, give us a shout!

Step 2: Practice

After you've taken the time to plan and prepare for your interview, now is the time to practice.

Practice Alone

You know how to study already. Consider your interview one of the most important tests of your life and plan accordingly. It is important to not just read the material but speak it too. Try recording your answers and then going back and listening to yourself. Do you sound fluid? Confident? Are you stammering or pausing inappropriately? Stand in front of a mirror and watch yourself. How do you look? Practice making eye contact. Practice until you are comfortable with your answers.

Also, practice as if it were the actual interview. Wear your interview outfit. Try sitting upright and even standing. You will not be interviewing while slouching on the couch or lying in bed. Just like athletes, the more accurately you reproduce the event in advance, the better prepared you will be.

It doesn't hurt to prepare mentally as well. Think about the interview. Imagine yourself answering confidently. You have come this far! Be confident! You can succeed!

Practice With Others

If you have a supportive family, friends, or even a tutor, they can help you prepare as well. After practicing alone, give them your questions and have them randomly ask you questions. While they might not know the exact answer, they will be able to assess your presentation of the information. Just talking to an actual person will increase your anxiety and that will help you perform better! The more you practice doing this, the easier it gets.

If your help is willing, recruit three or four people and have them conduct a mock panel interview. Wear your interview outfit. Have your group ask your questions with different wording. Record the experience. Then analyze the material. Where did you falter? How can your improve? Practice leads to success!

Step 3: Perform

After all your practice, the day will come when you have the interview. The school is talking to you because the faculty feels you may be a good fit for that school. They believe you may be the one they want! Thus, if you attend an interview, you will probably be either waitlisted or accepted unless you lied or cheated on the application, or unless you totally blew the interview.

Make sure you have your own questions answered. While they are evaluating you, you are also evaluating their school as well. This is your big moment!

Finally, as your complete your interviews, continue to use *Chart 1: Application & Interview Tracking* to record your interview results. After the interview, were you accepted? Waitlisted? Keeping track of all your information in one place will help you make decisions at a later date.

Mrs. C's Tips: Faking It

Fake it until you make it is popular saying that Mrs. C agrees with 100%. Even today after years of teaching and addressing large groups of students in the classroom, if she has a crucial presentation for an educational conference or her own job interview, you'll find her in an empty classroom practicing the presentation with the available technology, dressed in her suit speaking to empty chairs. Why? Practice makes perfect, or at the least, it makes for excellence. The more you practice your interview questions in your interview outfit, the better you'll be. Even if you are nervous during the interview, you can present well if you practice. For Lucas' interview practice, we set up a small panel of interviewers, asking him original questions based on the ones he prepared. Even if you're on your own in your practice, you can still have an audience. Use your phone to record yourself and evaluate how you make eye contact, how you convey meaning through body language, and how you sound. If you want to do well in your interview, practice, practice, practice!

CHAPTER 6: PREPARE ALTERNATIVE ROUTES
After December

After your interviews, there are three possible outcomes: being accepted, being rejected, or being waitlisted. If you are one of the many applicants who has been rejected or waitlisted, this chapter offers suggestions for your next steps.

You are likely disheartened right now. You have been working so hard, yet haven't succeeded here in this all important task. Yes, you knew it would be difficult, but you truly believed you would get in. Yet you didn't, so here you are. You have to accept the reality that not everyone who applies to medical school will get in. According to the AAMC, over 50% of medical school applicants will not get into a program the first time they apply. More than 50%! If you are in that category, you are not alone.

Maybe you know for sure you haven't been accepted, or maybe you are sitting, hoping against hope that you will get in. Regardless, you don't have to wait until the end of the cycle to anticipate the results. While schools rarely inform you directly that you haven't been accepted, using a silent rejection instead, you don't have to sit and wonder what is happening. For the most part, since medical schools follow the application timeline we have indicated, you can predict, to some extent, where you stand in the process.

Timeline Predictions	
For the Secondary Application:	If it's July to August and you haven't received a secondary application, you **probably** won't.
For the Interview:	If it's December and you haven't received an interview request, you **probably** won't.
After the Interview:	If several months have passed and you haven't been accepted or rejected, you **probably** will be waitlisted and your acceptance will depend on where you are on the waitlist; you may not get accepted this cycle.

* We say **probably** as there is always the slim chance that the school is either running behind or has some spots open at the last minute.

Mrs. C's Tips: Understanding the Waitlist

On the upside, if you are waitlisted, you can be pleased that the school does want you as a student; it is better than being rejected outright. Because there are a limited number of available spots, you are just at the bottom of the list, but at least you on the list. If you are at the top of the waitlist, say at number five or above, you have a good chance of moving up the list and getting accepted if other students decline to attend that school, which will free up enrollment spots. If, however, you are towards the bottom of the waitlist, say number fifteen or below, then your chances are not as good because fifteen applicants would have to decline to attend the school before you would have a chance at admittance. Every school has its own projected outcomes based on how many students they accepted and waitlisted. Nonetheless, there is still an opportunity for acceptance. On the downside, now you have to just wait for others to decide what they will do as those decisions will affect your future. This uncertainty can be nerve-racking, to say the least. Nonetheless, even in this unsettling situation, you can have an impact on your future. In the school's waitlisted notification, you will have been given a contact number for questions. You should call that school to inquire about your status and what they anticipate the outcome from the waitlist to be. Some schools move many students through their waitlist, but others don't. Lucas was fortunate as he had been accepted to other schools as well as being ranked 11th at the University of Iowa, Carver College of Medicine, where he ultimately chose to attend after moving up the waitlist into being accepted by the school. We suggest you follow the steps in Route One as much as possible as you wait to see what happens. While you may not have time to take a class, you can absolutely get more medical experience. Prepare yourself to reapply, just in case that is your only option.

The possible scenarios applicants find themselves in are endless. Perhaps you have had no interviews, so it has been made clear to you that this is not your year. Perhaps you have had many interviews and are waitlisted at several schools. In this situation, you still have a chance to get it so you may choose to hope and wait. Regardless, at this point, you are most likely asking yourself why you are in this situation and what you should do now. You need to take a hard look at your application process. Maybe you know exactly why you didn't get accepted, or maybe you have no idea. Review the following three most common reasons that students don't get accepted to medical school.

Common Reasons for Non-acceptance	
1.	Scores were not competitive. If your MCAT score or GPA is below average amongst those applying, you are not in a strong position. An MCAT of 32 (510 NEW) or lower or a GPA of 3.7 or lower may not be strong enough for your acceptance.
2.	Applications were weak in some area. If your essay or activities are poorly written with grammar errors and vague examples, if you lack an obvious connection to medicine through out-of-class experience or research, or if you only submitted the minimum required letters of recommendations or activities, then you were not in a strong position.
3.	Application materials were not submitted promptly or were missing materials. If you waited too long to submit your primary or secondary applications, then you were not in a strong position.

Take some time and be honest with yourself. Put aside the rejection and the hurt. Be objective about your application and your actions during the process. Where were your weaknesses? Where were your strengths? Then, ask yourself:

Why Didn't I Get Accepted?

If you are in this situation now, what should your next course of action be? You basically have two possible routes: Improve Your Application or Change Your Expectations. We will go into depth for both of these choices.

Mrs. C's Tips: Embrace Your Weakness

So you didn't get in despite all your hard work and effort. You are frustrated and discouraged. Take a minute and explore those feelings – they are valid and real. Now, recognize your weakness in this process and don't be afraid of it. Others will see it, so you might as well draw attention to it. Not getting into medical school feels like an ultimate failure for you right now; however, keep in mind the majority of students don't get in the first time. Make sure you explain what you've done to improve for the next application cycle. You can turn this weakness into a strength that actually propels your to excellence for next year's cycle! It's not easy to do that, but you must if you want to be successful. You can do this!

Route One: Improve Your Application

Simply reapplying next cycle with the same data you have thus far could very well result in the same result: non-acceptance. Therefore, you need to improve your application. Try and look at your application experience as objectively as you can and assess where you have room for improvement. We encourage you not only to address any obvious errors you may have had, such as a low MCAT score but to also add other more subtle improvements as well. The more areas in which you can improve the application, the more competitive you will be, thus more likely to get accepted next cycle. Consider the following suggestions for actions you can take to better reapply next cycle.

Retake MCAT	
Study Alone	Get MCAT books and study.
Take a Class	Take MCAT classes at Princeton Review, Kaplan, or other test prep.
Get a Tutor	Hire a private tutor for specific areas of weakness.
Complete all of the above if you want to do the best you can. Here is one area that improvement will make a huge difference in your future application, so do whatever it takes to improve the MCAT score.	
Improve GPA	
Take a Class	Take science and math classes at a community college.
Take a Program	Enroll in a Postbac program.
Your science and math grades need to be high to be a doctor. You won't last in medical school if you don't have the appropriate background, so take the time now to learn what you need to know.	

Improve Activities

Get Medical Activities	Find a physician to work with or volunteer in a medical environment.
Get Non-Medical Activities	Tutor/ teach a class or complete research.

Out-of-class activities are must haves to be competitive in the application process. Medical related activities are the most beneficial, so you should focus on those first.

Improve Letters of Recommendation

Get Better Letters	Get both science and non-science instructor letters. Get nonacademic letters, especially medical related references.
Provide More Letters	Provide the maximum number of letters allowed for each application.

The new experiences you've been acquiring in improving your scores and activities should give you additional resources for letters of recommendation.

Improve Written Work

Spend More Time	Spend more time on your responses for the essay and activity section.
Get Help	Engage a tutor or editor to help you with the written portions.

The primary application essay partially gets you the secondary responses. The secondary activities partially get you the interview. Thus, improving these sections improved your chances for admittance.

Improve School Choices

Choose Better	Choose appropriate STANDARD and SAFETY schools.
Apply to More	Choose more appropriate schools for which you qualify.

By only choosing those schools where your scores qualify you and applying to as many as you can, you will be more competitive and more successful.

Improve Application Timeline

Submit Primary Earlier	Apply as early as possible in the application cycle.
Submit Secondary Faster	Return your completed secondaries within three days of receipt.

Being first in line demonstrates organization and provides more chances for interviews.

Improve Interview Skills

Prepare More	Spend more time and energy preparing for your interviews.
Get Help	Engage someone to help you prepare.
Interview More	Attend every interview offered.

Polishing your interview skills should help you in this process How you conduct yourself in the interview may determine whether you get waitlisted or accepted.

We would suggest that you do as many of the Improve Your Application steps as you can before you reapply. Of course, in addition to those steps, you can go through this guide again. Doubtless, there are sections that you skipped or advice you didn't follow. This time, be more meticulous in your preparation. When you reapply, you will be answering the secondary questions about what you have done to improve yourself for the new application. Make sure you spend the time to write a good response for that section. Be prepared to show great effort! Be sure and use *Checklist 11: Reapply Preparation* in Chapter 9: Utilize Checklists to help you organize your activities.

> *Mrs. C's Tips: Get Help*
>
> *One of the characteristics of having excellence is to acknowledge when your own effort alone is not enough to result in a successful outcome. Sometimes to triumph one has to get help. For better or worse, such assistance may involve a financial outlay. Even though MCAT classes and private tutoring are expensive, in the long run, they may be cheaper than not getting accepted into medical school. You have to balance cost and time to decide what you can actually afford.*

Route Two: Change Your Expectations

Becoming an MD is one of the hardest tasks in academia today. As we have seen, simply being accepted into a medical school is a great achievement. If you find yourself to be one of the many students who simply can't get admitted to a medical school program, this does not mean you can't have a career in medicine. Being an MD is not the only possible choice; many other legitimate, necessary, and ultimately fulfilling medical professions are available as well.

Below are summarized some of the possible alternatives to an MD program. Each has its own positive and negative aspects. If you are interested in one of those programs, do some research. Go to the given website. Investigate if this could be a path for you. If you do apply to one of those programs, much of the information about the personal statement and application as well as the information about interviewing can help you with any future application you may submit.

Consider an Osteopathic Program.

A Doctor of Osteopathic Medicine (DO) is a licensed physician who practices all areas of medicine, but who emphasizes a whole-person approach to medicine. While these are rigorous programs, the GPA and MCAT score requirements for DO programs are generally lower than those of MD programs. For more information, go to the American Association of Colleges of Osteopathic Medicine at www.aacom.org.

Consider a Podiatrist Program.

A Doctor of Podiatric Medicine (DPM) is a licensed physician, specializing in the prevention, diagnosis and treatment of foot disorders resulting from injury or disease. While these are rigorous programs, the GPA and MCAT score requirements for DPM programs are generally lower than those of MD programs. For more information, go to the Council of Podiatric Medicine at http://www.cpme.org/index.cfm.

Consider an Optometrist Program.

A Doctor of Optometry is a licensed physician who diagnoses and treats vision problems. Instead of the MCAT, to get into an optometry program, the Optometry Admissions Test (OAT) is required. While these are rigorous programs, they may be less competitive than MD programs. For more information, go to the Association of Schools and Colleges of Optometry at http://www.opted.org/ or the American Optometric Association at http://www.aoa.org/.

Consider a Dental Program.

A Doctor of Dental Science (DDS) or a Doctor of Dental Medicine (DMD) is a licensed dentist who provides preventive and restorative treatments for problems affecting the mouth and teeth. Instead of the MCAT, to get into a dental program, the Dental Admission Test (DAT) is required. While these are rigorous programs, they may be less competitive than MD programs. For more information, go to the American Dental Education Association at http://www.adea.org.

Consider a Pharmacy Program.

A Doctor of Pharmacy (Pharm.D.) is a licensed professional who prepares, dispenses, and controls medications. Instead of the MCAT, to get into a pharmacy program the Pharmacy College Admission Test (PCAT) is required. While these are rigorous programs, they may be less competitive than MD programs. For more information, go to American Association of Colleges of Pharmacy at http://www.aacp.org/.

Consider an EMS Program.

Emergency Medical Services (EMS) include Emergency Medical Responders, Emergency Medical Technicians, and Paramedics. The requirements vary state by state. While these are rigorous programs, they may be less competitive than MD programs. For more information, go to the National Association of Medical Technicians at www.naemt.org.

Consider a Physician's Assistant Program.

A Physician's Assistant practices medicine under the supervision of an MD. The requirements and schools vary from state to state. While these are rigorous programs, they may be less competitive than MD programs. You can find more information from the American Academy of Physician's Assistants at www.aapa.org.

Consider a Public Health Career.

A Master's in Public Health offers many avenues to help others medically and could be a good choice for you as well. Some of the career possibilities with an MPH are Biosecurity Specialist, Bioterrorism Researcher, Chief Medical Officer, Clinical Infectious Disease Specialist, just to name a few. There are simply too many programs to give a website reference, but if you are interested, there will be something in your area.

We have offered two differing routes to review if you do not get into this year's cycle. Remember, this is not a defeat, but a normal process since the acceptance rate is so low the first year. Don't be discouraged and don't give up. You have come this far! Now is the time to re-evaluate what it is you really want. Ask yourself, why did you want to practice medicine in the first place? Then you can decide which of the two routes is best for you!

Mrs. C's Tips: Changing a Dream

Changing direction is not the same as giving up. In actuality, often times in life we are compelled to change our directions in unanticipated ways. When I was in school, I had planned to follow the traditional instructor path to earn a Ph.D., obtain a college tenure-track position, and teach happily ever after; that particular path did not work out for me. Nonetheless, here I am, not a failure despite not having a Ph.D. or tenure-track position. I am successfully teaching at various colleges, and perhaps more importantly, I am helping you succeed through this book. I am living my teaching dream even though it is not the one I initially designed, and I'm exceedingly happy with the direction I have found. Don't be afraid to change direction if required! You can succeed!

CHAPTER 7: PREPARE TO SUCCEED

The process is over – you have been accepted into one or more schools and are getting ready to go to medical school! Congratulations!

How now should you prepare for success? The first and most important factor is choosing the best school for you. Then, you must plan to handle the extreme, varied stresses of medical school itself.

If you have received multiple offers from various schools, you will want to consider many factors regarding which school will be the best choice for you. Most importantly, the academic environment of the school, as it will affect you personally, should be analyzed. All schools will provide an intense program of study, but based on your own history, one may be better for you than another. Succeeding in a medical program will most likely be the most difficult thing you have ever endeavored, so consider the following five factors when deciding which school to attend. These techniques should aid you in choosing wisely.

Choose Stress

Through this application process, you should have discovered a lot about yourself and what you want to accomplish. While keeping in mind every level of medical school will be very stressful, you can choose the stress level that you think will be most conducive to your career goals.

STRETCH schools will present the highest stress situations. The students you attend classes with may be more advanced than you in knowledge and experience so you will have to work that much harder to compete in that environment. Nonetheless, you are certainly able to do so, or the school wouldn't have accepted you! Just be aware that this will be a super challenging environment for you.

STANDARD schools will present the average amount of medical school stress situations. Your experience and grades have put you solidly in the middle of the pack. While still competitive, you may be average in your class and so may be under less pressure here. You can strive and be at the top of your class with hard work and determination. You can be quite accomplished in this environment!

SAFETY schools will present the least amount of stress comparatively. Coming in at the top of your class, your grades and experience should make you a leader. You can be a driving force in your program. Realize that while attending any medical school will be stressful, attending here may give you the best chance of success if you have other extenuating circumstances. You can thrive in this environment!

Choose School Program

Another thing to consider is the school's programs. Every medical school will have something to aid you in becoming a physician. The key is to decide which one will fit in best with your specific goals.

School Programs will differ from school to school. While every school will have similar medical basic training, the specific program in one school over another could affect your decision. For example, if you think you're interested in pediatrics, then one school might have a better possibility for this specialty than another. Hence, understanding what you're interested in is what will help you make these decisions.

Size and location of different schools will vary and create diverse situations. For example, the Medical College of Wisconsin, #36 on *Chart 4: School Selection Statistics* is a small private college. In comparison, the University of Iowa, #89 is a large state school. It's reasonable to assume that the environments of the two schools would differ greatly as well as the patient population and possibly even the diseases and conditions treated there. Similarly, a large urban University like UCLA #77 could be extremely different than either Wisconsin or Iowa. You should thus consider the environment of the school when choosing between possible choices.

Choose Finances

Money is obviously an important overall factor. All medical programs are expensive, and you will undoubtedly be taking on loans just to attend; however, not all programs are equally expensive. Some programs might cost more than others, and some schools will offer varying financial aid packages. The overall cost of living, not to mention out-of-state tuition, will differ as well. When deciding between three excellent out-of-state colleges, the financial aid package offered by each school factored into Lucas' decision as to where to attend. When looking at school choices, consider all the financial ramifications of your decision.

Choose Physical Environment

Weather may factor into your decision as well. Even within the same state, you may have environmental differences that affect you. The weather in sunny San Diego is quite different from that in foggy San Francisco. If you are moving out of state, the different weather could greatly affect you. For example, Lucas moved from Southern California into the heart of the Midwest, Iowa. Winter weather was a new experience complete with below zero temperatures and snow storms. He chose that school despite the weather, but he did think about it a bit!

Location may be a factor for you as well. You may have to move out of your comfort zone. You may be giving up environmental factors that are important to you. Many aspects of life are affected by where something is. Big city versus small town. Driving versus public transportation. Think about the size of the city and the availability of transportation as you evaluate each school.

Choose Lifestyle

Lifestyle could be a factor as well. In reality, most of your time will be consumed by the academic course load itself; nonetheless, every school in every state has its own culture. Possible recreational activities differ from school to school. Food availability may differ; general cultural considerations like music or clothing can affect your overall experience. Whether or not you can visit your family on a regular basis might matter to you, or perhaps if your family is moving with you, you will need to consider their needs as well. Even factors in the school that don't seemingly affect the medical school could affect the environment. Think about these things too.

You're going to spend some of the most formative years of your life and your career at the school that you choose now. Consider the factors we have suggested. Also, consider other factors that may apply to your specific situation. Take time to think about it and make the best decision you can. You can use *Checklist 13: Final School Choice* in Chapter 9: Utilize Checklists to help you decide.

Mrs. C's Tips: Choose Carefully

If you are fortunate, you will have the opportunity to choose between schools. With such choice comes added pressure, however. Lucas was willing to attend any of the schools where he applied and with the first acceptance, we were ecstatic with the result. Then he received additional acceptances, and the choice became more complicated. Ultimately, he considered all the factors we've discussed and picked the best school for his future plans. You can do the same! Choose wisely!

CHAPTER 8: BE PROSPEROUS

As we finish up this book, Lucas is finishing his 1st year in medical school. It's been a wonderful, yet stressful ride. Based on his experience this far and Mrs. C's experience teaching college students, we have just a bit of final advice for your success. We won't be advising you how to study. If you've made it this far, you know how to study. Instead, we offer a few overall recommendations that you might not have thought of think of.

Manage Your Stress

Without a doubt, going to medical school will be one of the most difficult things, if not the most difficult thing, you've ever done. Managing your stress in this environment will be difficult but critical for your success. You will be studying most of the time. Despite this intense study environment, to be successful, make sure that you eat healthily. It will be tempting to simply eat what's convenient; however, your body is your instrument, and you need to take care of it. Similarly, make sure that you get as much sleep as possible. On average, Lucas currently only gets 4 to 5 hours of sleep a night. More would be better for his health, but less would be a disaster for his study. As much as you can take care of yourself. Finally, try and relax. Find something to do that enables you to relax whether it's practicing yoga, watching movies, face booking friends, whatever works for you. You won't have much time for these activities, but try and make some time.

Use Available Resources

Every medical school will have resources for you to enable your success. We highly suggest that you use any extra tutoring offered. Lucas' school puts the students into houses, rather like Hogwarts, to encourage camaraderie and teamwork. Not all schools do that, however. Your school will have various programs in place for your success. At the colleges where Mrs. C teaches, there is always free tutoring and counseling. The tutoring can come in handy if you get stuck on a topic. The counseling can help when you are overwhelmed beyond belief. Your school will have resources to help you succeed as well. Use them as much as you can!

Have Realistic Expectations

You have been an above average student up to this point, or you wouldn't have come this far. Be aware that now you will be in classes where everyone is above average. Many people will be smarter than you, more organized than you, more popular than you, and so on. You have to be realistic about what you can and can't achieve. You may not be at the top of your class every time. You may even fail a test.

Lucas failed his first college test ever this year. He was studying for one important test and neglected to spend enough time to study for a test in another class. He bombed that test. He was distraught, to say the least, and had to regroup and rearrange his study time to give him enough time for the second class as well. With his new plan, he managed to do well in the class and finish it with an A. Nonetheless, it was a very stressful experience.

If you are doing your best that is all you can do. Be practical and pragmatic when it comes to what you expect in medical school. There will be huge disappointments, but also fantastic gratification as well!

Plan Short-Term Goals

Make plans for the current calendar, of course, but also think ahead to short term goals. For example, once you start school, look for opportunities that may arise for the summer. There will be internships or teaching opportunities that you have to prepare for. In your first semester, you should be planning for your second. In your second, for summer. During the summer, you should be planning for the upcoming year. Don't just think about your daily goals and weekly goals. Of course, you need those! Nonetheless, you will also need to think beyond the immediacy for the short-term too.

Preserve Long-Term Goals

You wanted to be a doctor for a reason. Keep that reason in mind during the stressful, overwhelming days of study and preparation. Dream about your future practice, where it will be and what it will look like. Think about how you will treat your patients. The day or days will come where you think that you can't do this anymore or that you won't ever be a doctor. Lucas has been the most focused, driven student that Mrs. C has ever worked with, yet even he has had days of defeat when he thought he couldn't complete this difficult course. Attending medical school is an intense, stressful pressure cooker with so many things to learn in such a short amount of time. Hold on to those long-term goals that you set out to accomplish. Don't be afraid to change them as necessary as you learn more details about the actual practice of medicine, but don't, ever, give up on your dreams!

It's been an exciting journey for you getting here thus far. There's been pleasure and there's been pain. We're sure that your journey has been fraught with peril and brought extreme joy.

Thank you for purchasing and reading our guide to the medical school application process. We'd love to hear from you about your journey, about your experience in the application process, about your response to the book, or even about your time in medical school.

If you want to chat with Lucas about med school or Mrs. C about the book, they would love to hear from you. You can find them on Facebook at www.facebook.com/medicalschoolapplication. If you are interested in getting help with your personal statement or some of your responses, you can ask about her private editing or tutoring rate. You can also email Mrs. C directly at classroom@clmn.net.

We both wish you the best as you pursue your new fabulous, fantastic career in medicine!

Mrs. C's Tips: Enjoy the Journey

You've chosen a highly competitive career in seeking to become a physician. While helping others can be a highly rewarding endeavor, practicing medicine in America is also filled with paperwork and malpractice insurance. Doctors often see people at their worst in the most difficult moments of their lives. Therefore, we encourage you to enjoy the journey as you strive to meet your goals. Take time to relax and have a bit of fun now and again. Try as much as possible to have balance in your life. Life is fleeting, so make the most of every minute!

CHAPTER 9: UTILIZE CHECKLISTS

We understand how overwhelming the process can be. With so many details, it is easy to overlook something important, causing delays or rejections. Thus, we have provided itemized checklists for each stage of the application process so that you can have one place for all your relevant information. You will find the checklists in the order detailed below. Each is designed to accompany a specific aspect of the guide. We have organized them in such a way that you can cut them out to carry with you if you find that helpful as well.

By utilizing the checklists, you can be sure that you have not forgotten a vital detail.

Checklist 1: Readiness to Apply

Checklist 2: Recommendation Letters Overall

Checklist 3: Recommendation Letters Itemized

Checklist 4: Personal Statement

Checklist 5: My School Choices

Checklist 6: School Selection Overall

Checklist 7: Primary Application Preparation

Checklist 8: Secondary Application Preparation

Checklist 9: Interview Responses Preparation

Checklist 10: Interview Overall Planning

Checklist 11: Reapply Preparation

Checklist 12: Alternative Choices

Checklist 13: Final School Choice

Checklist 14: Create Your Own

Checklist 1: Readiness to Apply

Are My Scores Sufficient?

☐ Did I Take My MCAT 1.5 Months In Advance Of Applying?

☐ Are My MCAT Score & GPA Above Average? MCAT *32 (Or 511) & 3.7 GPA?*

 MCAT Score Is_____ Overall GPA Is _____ Science GPA Is _____

☐ If Not, Can One Of The Scores Compensate For The Other?
 *No Lower Than 30 (508) On MCAT Regardless Of Both GPA
 *No Lower Than 3.7 On Both GPA Unless MCAT Is Higher Than 38 (519)

2. Have I Earned An Appropriate Degree?

☐ *My Degree Is _____*

Do I Have Volunteer Experience?

☐ Have I Volunteered In A Medical Institution For At Least 6 Months?

☐ Have I Completed Other Medical-related Volunteer Activities?

☐ Have I Completed Non-medical Volunteer Activities?

Have I Completed Any Research?

☐ *My Research Is _____*

Have I Accumulated Any Unique Experiences?

☐ *My Unique Experience Is_____*

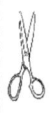

Checklist 2: Recommendation Letters Overall

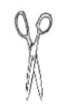

For My Recommender Choices:

☐   Did I Earn An A In That Class?

☐   Does The Writer Know Me Well?

☐   Has The Writer Known Me A Long Time? How Long?

☐   Have I Shown Extraordinary Ability Or Effort For The Writer?

☐   Will The Writer Tailor The Letter For Medical School?

☐   Can I Have A Personal Copy Of The Letter?

For My Actual Letters, Do I Have The:

☐   Two Required Academic Science Recommendations?

☐   One Required Academic Non-Science Recommendation?

☐   MD Optional Recommendation?

☐   Research Optional Recommendation?

☐   Medical Volunteer Optional Recommendation?

☐   Academic Work Optional Recommendation?

☐   General Volunteer Optional Recommendation?

☐   Work Optional Recommendation?

☐   Unique-To-Me Optional Recommendation?

Checklist 3: Recommendation Letters Itemized

#	Requested From	Date Requested	Date Received

Checklist 4: Personal Statement

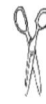

In My Personal Statement, Do I Clearly State:

☐ Reason For Med School?

☐ Medical Exposure?

☐ Academic Preparedness?

☐ Work Experience?

☐ Leadership Experience?

☐ Unique Experiences?

☐ Personal Strengths?

☐ Long - Term Goals?

In My Personal Statement, Did I Carefully Check:

☐ Structural Format?

☐ Word Choices?

☐ Grammar Usage?

☐ Punctuation Usage?

Checklist 5: My School Choices

Standard Schools

1	11	21
2	12	22
3	13	23
4	14	24
5	15	25
6	16	26
7	17	27
8	18	28
9	19	29
10	20	30

Safety Schools

1	3	5
2	4	

Stretch Schools

1	3	5
2	4	

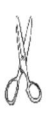

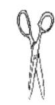

Checklist 6: School Selection Overall

Did I Select:

- ☐ All My State's Schools? ** If My Scores Were Sufficient*
- ☐ 20-30 Standard Schools?
- ☐ 5 Stretch Schools?
- ☐ 5 Safety Schools?
- ☐ Minimum of 40 Total Schools?

Checklist 7: Primary Application Preparation

Did I Complete, Verify, And Review:

- ☐ Identifying Information?
- ☐ School Information?
- ☐ Biographic Information?
- ☐ Course Work?
- ☐ Activity List?
- ☐ Letters Of Evaluation?
- ☐ Medical School Selection?
- ☐ Personal Statement Essay?
- ☐ Standardized Test Scores?

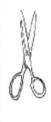

Checklist 8: Secondary Application Preparation

Did I Write Polished Paragraphs For:

- ☐ Autobiographical Uniqueness?
  - ☐ My Reason To Choose Medicine
  - ☐ My Experiences With Team Work
  - ☐ My Achievements
- ☐ Diversity Experience?
  - ☐ My Experiences With Diversity
  - ☐ My Value A School's Diversity
- ☐ Postbac Activities?
  - ☐ My Activities Since Graduation
- ☐ Challenging Situations
  - ☐ My Obvious Weakness
  - ☐ My Overcome Obstacle / Failure
- ☐ Future Plans?
  - ☐ My Future In 5, 10, 15 Years
  - ☐ My General Plans
- ☐ School Specific?
  - ☐ Specific Programs Or Environmental Interests
- ☐ Other?
  - ☐ Specific Explainable Weakness

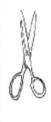

Checklist 9: Interview Responses Preparation

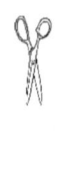

Have I Planned My Words For Excellent Response To The:

☐ Personal Characteristic - Personal Background Questions?

☐ Personal Characteristic - Individual Characteristic Questions?

☐ Personal Characteristic - Thought Process Questions?

☐ Personal Characteristic - Acquired Activity Questions?

☐ Personal Characteristic - Overcoming Adversity Questions?

☐ Healthcare Issue - You Questions?

☐ Healthcare Issue - Community Questions?

☐ Healthcare Issue - World Questions?

☐ Medical Scenario Questions?

☐ School Specific Questions?

For My Questions About The Specific School, Have I:

☐ Reviewed The Given Questions?

☐ Asked The Questions In Various Ways?

☐ Created My Own Relevant Questions?

Checklist 10: Interview Overall Planning

☐ **Have I Adequately Planned My Interview Responses?**

Have I Budgeted Adequately For:

☐ Look?

☐ Transportation?

☐ Lodging?

☐ Food?

☐ Time?

☐ Money?

Have I Planned An Appropriate Look For My:

☐ Head?

☐ Top?

☐ Bottom?

☐ Toes?

☐ Accessories?

Have I Planned Travel For My:

☐ Transportation?

☐ Lodging?

☐ Food?

☐ Campus Activities?

☐ Weather?

☐ Technology?

Checklist 11: Reapply Preparation

Have I...

☐   Improved My MCAT Score?

☐   Improved My GPA?

☐   Improved My Activities?

☐   Improved My Recommendation Letters?

☐   Improved My Written Work?

☐   Improved My School Choices?

☐   Improved My Application Timeline?

☐   Improved My Interviewing Skills?

Checklist 12: Alternative Choices

Should I Consider:

☐   An Osteopathic Program? (www.aacom.org)

☐   A Podiatrist Program? (http://www.cpme.org/index.cfm)

☐   An Optometrist Program? (http://www.opted.org)

☐   A Dental Program? (http://www.adea.org)

☐   A Pharmacy Program? (http://www.aacp.org)

☐   An EMS Program? (www.naemt.org)

☐   A Physician's Assistant Program? (www.aapa.org)

☐   A Public Health Program?

Checklist 13: Final School Choice

For the Schools I've Been Accepted to, Have I Considered...

☐ My Stress Level?

☐ School Programs?

☐ School Financial Packages?

☐ School Physical Environment?

☐ School Lifestyle?

My School Choice Is:

_____

Checklist 14: Create Your Own

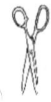

CHAPTER 10: UTILIZE CHARTS

These charts were actually the impetus for this guide; the charts started it all. As Lucas pursued his own application process, we looked all over the market for help. Unfortunately, most of the information was scattered here and there, so it was difficult to use. As we gathered the data needed for his application, we made charts with the only intent to fulfill his own dream of getting into medical school. The process took so much time and effort! Ultimately, it resulted in his acceptance into four schools, so we were successful!

At some point during Lucas' application year, Mrs. C took two new private students who were applying to medical school. Lucas graciously gave permission to use the formulas and data created for his own process and with that, the book idea was born.

We have verified all the data as much as possible, but you must be aware that things are always changing, and the data in all the charts has been collected from various sources which themselves may have errors. Moreover, the new MCAT scoring will undoubtedly cause some changes we have not anticipated. Nonetheless, this information should provide sufficient information to will help you in your quest to get accepted to medical school! We have also included the chart Lucas used to track his own secondary responses and interviews. We think you will find it useful.

Chart 1: Application and Interview Tracking

Chart 2: MCAT Old to New Score Conversion

Chart 3: MCAT Score to Percentile Conversion

Chart 4: School Selection Statistics

Chart 5: Secondary Application Question Codes

Chart 6: Secondary Application Questions

Chart 7: Practice Interview Questions

Chart 8: Enlarged Process Timeline

Chart 1: Application and Interview Tracking

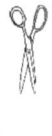

#	School	Received	Deadline	Submitted	ID and Password	Interview	Result
1							
2							
3							
4							
5							
6							
7							
8							
9							
10							
11							
12							
13							
14							
15							

#	School	Received	Deadline	Submitted	ID and Password	Interview	Result
17							
18							
19							
20							
21							
22							
23							
24							
25							
26							
27							
28							
29							
30							

#	School	Received	Deadline	Submitted	ID and Password	Interview	Result
32							
33							
34							
35							
36							
37							
38							
39							
40							
41							
42							
43							
44							
45							

Chart 2: MCAT Old to New Score Conversion

OLD	NEW	OLD	NEW	OLD	NEW
45	528	31	508	17	488
44	527	30	507	16	487
44	526	29	506	15	486
43	525	29	505	14	485
42	524	28	504	14	484
42	523	27	503	13	483
41	522	27	502	12	482
40	521	26	501	12	481
39	520	25	500	11	480
39	519	24	499	10	479
38	518	24	498	9	478
37	517	23	497	9	477
37	516	22	496	8	476
36	515	22	495	7	475
35	514	21	494	7	474
34	513	20	493	6	473
34	512	19	492	5	472
33	511	19	491		
32	510	18	490		
32	509	17	489		

Chart 3: MCAT Score to Percentile Conversion

MCAT SCORE OLD	24	30	33	36	39	45
MCAT SCORE NEW	500	308	512	516	520	528
PERCENTILE	50%	75%	90%	97%	99%	100%

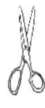

111

Chart 4: School Selection Statistics

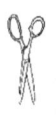

#	School				
	MCAT (OLD)	MCAT (NEW)	GPA ALL	GPA S	In-State
1	**Albany Medical College**				
	28 - 35	504- 514	3.29 - 3.89	3.09 - 3.89	N
2	**Albert Einstein**				
	31 - 37	508 - 517	3.56 - 3.96	3.49 – 3.98	N
3	**Baylor**				
	31 - 38	508 - 518	3.63 – 3.99	3.54 – 4.0	Y
4	**Boston University**				
	31 / 35 / 39	508 / 514 / 519-520	3.45 / 3.79 / 3.97	3.37 / 3.76 / 3.98	N
5	**Brown (Warren Alpert)**				
	28 / 33 / 37	504 / 511 / 516-517	3.41 / 3.75 / 3.96	3.2 / 3.73 / 3.99	N
6	**Case Western**				
	33 / 36 / 39	511 / 515 / 519-520	3.51 / 3.8 / 3.98	3.43 / 3.79 / 3.98	N
7	**Central Michigan**				
	27 / 32 / 36	502-503 / 509-510 / 515	3.43 / 3.71 / 3.92	3.25 / 3.63 / 3.91	Y
8	**Columbia**				
	23 / 36 / 40	497 / 515 / 521	3.57 / 3.83 / 3.98	3.47 / 3.83 / 4	N
9	**Cornell (Weill)**				
	32 / 36 / 40	509 – 510 / 515 / 521	3.63 / 3.85 / .99	3.57 / 3.85 / 4	N
10	**Creighton University**				
	28 / 31 / 34	504 / 508 / 512-513	3.49 / 3.82 / 3.97	3.37 / 3.79 / 3.99	N
11	**Dartmouth (Geisel)**				
	30 /34 / 38	507 / 512-513 / 518	3.42 / 3.76/ 3.96	3.29 / 3.75 / 3.98	N
12	**Drexel University**				
	28 / 31 / 35	504 / 508 / 514	3.34 / 3.82 / 3.97	3.25 / 3.63 / 3.9	N
13	**Duke**				
	31 / 36 / 40	508 / 515 / 521	3.49 / 3.86 / 4.0	3.41 / 3.85 / 4.0	N
14	**East Carolina (Brody)**				
	26 / 30 / 34	501 / 507 / 512-513	3.24 / 3.72 / 3.95	3 / 3.69 / 3.96	Y
15	**East Tennessee (Quillen)**				
	25 / 29 / 34	500 / 505-506 / 512-513	3.43 / 3.76 / 3.96	3.28 / 3.72 / 3.97	Y
16	**Eastern Virginia**				
	28 / 32 / 36	504 / 509-510 / 515	3.29 / 3.66/ 3.91	3.15 / 3.61 / 3.94	Y
17	**Emory**				
	31 / 35 / 38	508 / 514 / 518	3.45 / 3.78 / 3.96	3.3 / 3.74 / 3.98	N
18	**Florida Atlantic**				
	29 / 33 / 36	505-506 / 511 / 515	3.34 / 3.71 / 3.97	3.21/3.67/3.96	Y

#	School				
	MCAT (OLD)	MCAT (NEW)	GPA ALL	GPA S	In-State
19	Florida International University				
	28 / 31 / 35	508 / 508 / 514	3.37 / 3.7 / 3.95	3.25 / 3.64 / 3.96	N
20	Florida State				
	24 / 29 / 33	498-499 / 505-506 / 511	3.37 / 3.71 / 3.97	3.28 / 3.68 / 3.98	Y
21	George Washington University				
	27 / 31 / 35	502-503 /508 / 514	3.48 / 3.74 / 3.93	3.3 / 3.68 / 3.93	N
22	Georgetown University				
	27 / 31 / 35	502-503 / 508 / 514	3.48 / 3.74 / 3.93	3.3 / 3.68 / 3.93	N
23	Harvard				
	32 / 37 / 41	509-510 / 516-517 / 522	3.73 / 3.93 / 4.0	3.73 / 3.94 / 4.0	N
24	Hofstra North Shore				
	30 / 33 / 37	507 / 511 / 516-517	3.41 / 3.68 / 3.91	3.28 / 3.63 / 3.93	N
25	Howard University				
	24 / 27 / 32	498-498 / 503-503 / 509-510	2.94 / 3.41 / 3.88	2.74 / 3.22 / 3.86	N
26	Indiana University				
	26 / 31 / 36	501 / 508 / 515	3.41 / 3.8 / 3.98	3.28 / 3.76 / 3.99	Y
27	Jefferson				
	29 / 32 /36	505-506 / 509-510 / 515	3.45 / 3.71 / 3.94	3.35 / 3.68 / 3.96	N
28	Johns Hopkins				
	32 / 36 / 40	509-510 / 515 / 521	3.7 / 3.91 / 4.0	3.69 / 3.91 / 4.0	N
29	Loma Linda				
	25 / 31 / 36	500 / 508 / 515	3.52 / 3.83 / 3.98	3.47 / 3.81 / 3.99	N
30	Loyola (Stritch)				
	29 / 33 / 37	505-506 / 511 / 516-517	3.37 / 3.72 / 3.95	3.27 / 3.69 / 3.98	N
31	LSU New Orleans				
	27 / 31 / 35	502-503 / 508 / 514	3.35 / 3.78 / 4.0	3.28 / 3.75 / 4.0	Y
32	LSU Shreveport				
	24 / 28 / 33	498-499 / 504 / 511	3.36 / 3.76 / 3.97	3.21 / 3.71 / 4.0	Y
33	Mayo Medical School				
	30 / 34 / 39	507 / 512-513 / 519-520	3.63 / 3.87 / 4	3.58 / 3.86 / 4.0	N
34	Marshall University (Edwards)				
	25 / 28 / 33	500 / 504 / 511	3.24 / 3.65 / 3.96	3.03 / 3.57 / 3.99	Y
35	Medical College Georgia				
	27 / 32 / 36	502-503 / 509-510 / 515	3.46 / 3.78 / 3.97	3.35 / 3.75 / 3.97	Y
36	Medical College Wisconsin				
	27 / 31 / 35	502-503 / 508 / 514	3.51 / 3.78 / 3.97	3.35 / 3.75 / 3.98	N

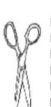

#	School				
	MCAT (OLD)	MCAT (NEW)	GPA ALL	GPA S	In-State
37	**Medical University of South Carolina**				
	25 / 31 / 36	500 / 508 / 515	3.24 / 3.72 / 3.98	3.09 / 3.67 / 4.0	Y
38	**Meharry Medical College**				
	24 / 27 / 30	498-499 / 502-503 / 507	3.2 / 3.52 / 3.88	3.03 / 3.41 / 3.88	N
39	**Mercer**				
	26 / 29 / 32	501 / 506 / 509-510	3.25 / 3.65 / 3.93	3.05 / 3.57 / 3.92	Y
40	**Michigan State**				
	25 / 30 / 34	500 / 507 / 512-513	3.19 / 3.68 / 3.94	3.05 / 3.58 / 3.93	Y
41	**Morehouse**				
	23 / 27 / 31	497 / 502-503 / 508	3.14 / 3.51 / 3.85	3 / 3.42 / 3.86	Y
42	**Mount Sinai (Icahn)**				
	33 /37 / 40	511 / 5166-517 / 521	3.6 / 3.85 / 3.98	3.47 / 3.85 / 4.0	N
43	**New York Medical College**				
	27 / 32 / 35	502-503 / 509-510 / 514	3.34 / 3.64 / 3.88	3.16 / 3.57 / 3.88	N
44	**NYU**				
	32 / 36 / 39	509-510 / 515 / 519-520	3.61 / 3.86 / 3.98	3.55 / 3.85 / 4.0	N
45	**Northwest Ohio**				
	24 / 28 / 32	498-499 / 504 / 509-510	3.44 / 3.77 / 3.97	3.27 / 3.75 / 3.99	Y
46	**Northwestern**				
	32 / 36 / 39	509-510 / 515 / 519-520	3.62 / 3.87 / 3.98	3.52 / 3.87 / 4	N
47	**Oakland University**				
	28 / 31 / 35	504 / 508 / 514	3.4 / 3.73 / 3.94	3.27 / 3.64 / 3.94	N
48	**Ohio State**				
	30 / 35 / 39	507 / 514 / 519-520	3.46 / 3.8 / 3.98	3.31 / 3.79 / 4.0	N
49	**Oregon Health & Science University**				
	28 / 32 / 36	504 / 509-510 / 515	3.33 / 3.76 / 3.95	3.3 / 3.73 / 3.97	Y
50	**Pennsylvania State University**				
	28 / 31 / 36	504 / 508 / 515	3.49 / 3.79 / 3.97	3.37 / 3.73 / 3.98	N
51	**Quinnipiac University (Netter)**				
	27 / 30 / 34	502-503 / 507 / 512-513	3.28 / 3.59 / 3.86	3.15 / 3.53 / 3.88	N
52	**Rosalind Franklin Chicago**				
	27 / 32 / 36	502 -503 / 509-510 / 515	3.38 / 3.79 / 3.96	3.31 / 3.78 / 3.98	Y
53	**Rowan University (Cooper)**				
	27 / 31 / 35	502-503 / 508 / 514	3.21 / 3.59 / 3.92	3.05 / 3.52 / 3.92	Y
54	**Rush Medical College**				
	28 / 31 / 34	504 / 508 / 512-513	3.43 / 3.65 / 3.92	3.24 / 3.58 / 3.92	N
55	**Rutgers University (NJMS)**				
	29 / 33 / 37	505 / 511 / 516-517	3.42 / 3.74 / 3.96	3.31 / 3.71 / 3.97	Y

#	MCAT (OLD)	MCAT (NEW)	GPA ALL	GPA S	In-State
		School			
56	Rutgers University (RWJMS)				
	29 / 33 / 37	505-506 / 511 / 516-517	3.35 / 3.72 / 3.96	3.22 / 3.65 / 3.98	Y
57	Saint Louis University				
	28 / 33 / 36	504 / 511 / 515	3.51 / 3.84 / 3.97	3.47 / 3.83 / 3.99	N
58	Southern Illinois University				
	25 / 30 / 35	500 / 507 / 514	3.2 / 3.73 / 3.99	2.97 / 3.69/ 4.0	Y
59	Stanford				
	33 / 37 / 41	511 / 516-517 / 522	3.61 / 3.85 / 3.99	3.53 / 3.85 / 4.0	N
60	Stony Brook				
	30 / 33 / 37	507 / 511 / 516-517	3.5 / 3.78 / 3.96	3.44 / 3.78 / 3.98	Y
61	SUNY Downstate				
	30 / 33 / 38	507 / 511 / 518	3.5 / 3.77 / 3.94	3.41 / 3.75 / 3.96	Y
62	SUNY Upstate				
	28 / 32 / 36	504 / 509-510 / 515	3.4 / 3.74 / 3.95	3.26 / 3.7 / 3.97	Y
63	Temple				
	29 / 32 / 35	505-506 / 509-510 / 514	3.46 / 3.73 / 3.95	3.34 / 3.68 / 3.95	N
64	Texas A&M				
	27 / 31 / 35	502-503 / 508 / 514	3.42 / 3.72 / 3.97	3.34 / 3.69 / 3.99	Y
65	Texas Tech (El Paso)				
	26 / 29 / 34	501 / 505-506 /512-513	3.46 / 3.77 / 3.97	3.32 / 3.72 / 3.99	Y
66	Common Wealth Med College				
	27 / 31 / 35	502/503 / 508 / 514	3.24 / 3.68 / 3.91	3.08 / 3.58 / 3.92	Y
67	Tufts				
	30 / 34 / 38	507 / 512-513 / 518	3.42 / 3.73 / 3.94	3.31 / 3.7 / 3.96	N
68	Tulane				
	31 / 33 / 36	508 / 511 / 515	3.27 / 3.61 / 3.9	3.12 / 3.51 / 3.91	N
69	Uniformed Services University				
	29 / 32 /35	506 / 509-510 / 514	3.34 / 3.66 / 3.93	3.26 / 3.62 / 3.93	N
70	University of Alabama				
	26 / 31 / 35	501 / 508 / 514	3.47 / 3.85 / 4.0	3.37 / 3.83 / 4.0	Y
71	University of Arizona (Tucson)				
	27 / 31 / 36	502-503 / 508 / 515	3.39 / 3.74 / 3.98	3.26 / 3.67 / 4.0	Y
72	University of Arizona (Phoenix)				
	27 / 31 / 36	502-503 / 508 / 515	3.37 / 3.76 / 3.99	3.33 / 3.73 / 4.0	Y
73	University of Arkansas				
	26 / 30 / 35	501 / 507 / 514	3.32 / 3.74 / 3.99	3.19 / 3.72 / 4.0	Y
74	University Buffalo State				
	27 / 32 / 36	503 / 509-510 / 515	3.49 / 3.75 / 3.95	3.37 / 3.73 / 3.95	Y

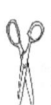

#	School				
	MCAT (OLD)	MCAT (NEW)	GPA ALL	GPA S	In-State
75	UC Davis				
	26 / 32 / 37	501 / 509-510 / 516-517	3.3 / 3.71 / 3.93	3.1 / 3.64 / 3.96	Y
76	UC Irvine				
	30 / 34 / 38	507 / 512-513 / 518	3.51 / 3.78 / 3.98	3.43 / 3.75 / 4.0	Y
77	UCLA				
	28 / 35 / 39	504 / 514 / 519-520	3.3 / 3.69 / 3.91	3.23 / 3.65 / 3.9	Y
78	UC Riverside				
	26 / 31 / 33	501 / 508 / 511	3.3 / 3.69 / 3.91	3.23 / 3.65 / 3.9	Y
79	UC San Diego				
	30 / 35 / 39	507 / 514 / 519 / 520	3.54 / 3.82 / 3.98	3.42 / 3.81 / 3.99	Y
80	UC San Francisco				
	31 / 36 / 40	508 / 515 / 421	3.57 / 3.85 / 3.99	3.5 / 3.86 / 4.0	Y
81	University of Central Florida				
	29 / 31 / 36	505 / 508 / 515	3.44 / 3.8 / 3.97	3.45 / 3.78 / 3.99	Y
82	University of Chicago (Pritzker)				
	33 /37 / 41	511 / 516-517 / 522	3.65 / 3.87 / 3.99	3.58 / 3.89 / 4.0	N
83	University of Cincinnati				
	30 / 34 / 38	507 / 512-513 / 518	3.35 / 3.78 / 3.98	3.24 / 3.72 / 3.99	N
84	University of Colorado				
	29 / 33 / 37	506 / 511 / 516-517	3.47 / 3.79 / 3.96	3.41 / 3.77 / 3.98	Y
85	University of Connecticut				
	28 / 33 / 37	504 / 511 / 516-517	3.51 / 3.79 / 3.96	3.44 / 3.79 / 3.98	Y
86	University of Florida				
	29 / 33 / 37	505-506 / 511 / 516-517	3.55 / 3.86 / 3.99	3.46 / 3.83 / 4.0	Y
87	University of Hawaii				
	27 / 31 / 36	502-503 / 508 / 515	3.38 / 3.78 / 3.97	3.26 / 3.74 / 3.98	Y
88	University of Illinois				
	26 / 32 / 37	501 / 509-510 / 516-517	3.26 / 3.7 / 3.96	3.1 / 3.64 / 3.97	Y
89	University of Iowa				
	29 / 33 / 37	506 / 511 / 516-517	3.48 / 3.84 / 3.98	3.42 / 3.81 / 4.0	Y
90	University of Kansas				
	24 /29 / 34	498-499 / 505-506 /511-512	3.41 / 3.77 / 3.99	3.28 / 3.74 / 4.0	Y
91	University of Kentucky				
	29 / 32 / 36	505-506 / 509-510 / 515	3.33 / 3.76 / 3.99	3.2 / 3.72 / 4.0	Y
92	University of Louisville				
	27 / 30 / 34	502-503 507 / 512-513	3.34 / 3.73 / 3.99	3.18 / 3.67 / 4.0	Y
93	University of Maryland				
	29 / 33 / 37	505-506 / 511 / 516-517	3.62 / 3.82 / 3.97	3.52 / 3.8 / 3.99	Y

#	School				
	MCAT (OLD)	MCAT (NEW)	GPA ALL	GPA S	In-State
94	University of Massachusetts				
	29 / 33 / 36	505-506 / 511 / 515	3.5 / 3.75 / 3.95	3.37 / 3.74 / 3.97	Y
95	University of Miami				
	30 / 32 / 36	507 / 209-510 / 515	3.43 / 3.77 / 3.98	3.27 / 3.72 / 3.99	N
96	University of Michigan				
	32 / 36 / 40	209-510 / 515 / 521	3.58 / 3.84 / 3.99	3.48 / 3.84 / 4.0	N
97	University of Minnesota				
	27 / 32 / 37	503 / 509-510 / 516-517	3.37 / 3.79 / 3.98	3.27 / 3.76 / 4.0	Y
98	University of Mississippi				
	24 / 28 / 33	498-499 / 504 / 511	3.23 / 3.76 / 4	3.1 / 3.7 / 4.0	Y
99	University of Missouri-Columbia				
	27 / 31 / 36	502-503 / 508 / 515	3.48 / 3.83 / 3.99	3.34 / 3.78 / 4.0	Y
100	University of Missouri-Kansas City				
	26 / 28 / 31	501 / 504 / 508	3.29 / 3.72 / 3.93	3.25 / 3.68 / 3.94	N
101	University of Nebraska				
	27 / 31 / 36	502-503 / 508 / 515	3.51 / 3.83 / 3.99	3.35 / 3.76 / 4.0	Y
102	University of Nevada				
	28 / 31 / 35	504 / 508 / 514	3.46 / 3.81 / 3.99	3.32 / 3.78 / 3.98	Y
103	University of New Mexico				
	23 / 28 / 33	497 / 504 / 511	3.18 / 3.66 / 3.95	3.02 / 3.58 / 3.95	Y
104	University of North Carolina				
	28 / 33 / 37	504 / 511 / 516-517	3.39 / 3.75 / 3.96	3.18 / 3.71 / 3.98	Y
105	University of North Dakota				
	24 / 29 / 35	498-499 / 505-506 / 514	3.39 / 3.74 / 3.97	3.14 / 3.67 / 4.0	Y
106	University of Oklahoma				
	27 / 31 / 35	502-503 / 508 / 514	3.52 / 3.84 / 4.0	3.38 / 3.79 / 4.0	Y
107	University of Pennsylvania (Raymond Ruth Perelman)				
	34 / 38 / 40	512-513 / 518 / 521	3.66 / 3.88 / 3.99	3.62 / 3.89 / 4	N
108	University of Pittsburgh				
	31 / 36 / 39	508 / 515 / 519-520	3.55 / 3.86 / 3.98	3.52 / 3.85 / 4.0	N
109	University of Rochester				
	29 / 34 / 38	505-506 / 512-513 / 518	3.55 / 3.77 / 3.96	3.41 / 3.74 / 3.98	N
110	University of South Alabama				
	27 / 30 / 35	502-503 / 507 / 514	3.52 / 3.86 / 4.0	3.35 / 3.83 / 4.0	Y
111	University of South Carolina Greenville				
	25 / 30 / 34	500 / 507 / 512-513	3.28 / 3.67 / 3.98	3.15 / 3.6 / 4.0	Y
112	University of South Carolina				
	25 / 31 / 36	500 / 508 / 515	3.24 / 3.72 / 3.98	3.09 / 3.67 / 4	Y

#	School				
	MCAT (OLD)	MCAT (NEW)	GPA ALL	GPA S	In-State
113	University of South Dakota (Sanford)				
	26 / 30 / 35	501 / 507 / 514	3.39 / 3.8 / 4.0	3.24 / 3.73 / 4.0	Y
114	University of South Florida				
	28 / 31 / 35	504 / 508 / 514	3.36 / 3.75 / 3.97	3.24 / 3.71 / 3.98	Y
115	USC				
	30 / 35 / 38	507 / 514 / 518	3.4 / 3.75 / 3.96	3.32 / 3.74 / 3.97	N
116	University of Tennessee				
	26 / 31 / 35	501 / 508 / 514	3.33 / 3.73 / 3.99	3.17 / 3.69 / 4.0	Y
117	University of Texas Medical Branch				
	28 / 32 / 36	504 / 509-510 / 515	3.42 / 3.76 / 3.98	3.26 / 3.71 / 3.99	Y
118	University of Texas Southwestern				
	31 / 35 / 38	508 / 514 / 518	3.63 / 3.87 / 4.0	3.53 / 3.87 / 4.0	Y
119	University of Toledo				
	28 / 32 / 36	504 / 509-510 / 515	3.42 / 3.82 / 3.98	3.26 / 3.79 / 3.99	Y
120	University of Utah				
	25 / 30 / 35	500 / 507 / 514	3.48 / 3.75 / 3.96	3.32 / 3.7 / 3.96	Y
121	University of Vermont				
	29 / 32 / 36	505-506 / 509-510 / 515	3.39 / 3.73 / 3.93	3.33 / 3.69 / 3.96	N
122	University of Virginia				
	32 / 36 / 39	509-510 / 515 / 519-520	3.51 / 3.87 / 3.99	3.43 / 3.87/ 4	N
123	University of Washington				
	27 / 31 / 38	502-503 / 508 / 518	3.4 / 3.73 / 3.97	3.2 / 3.69 / 3.98	N
124	University of Wisconsin				
	28 / 33 / 37	504 / 511 / 516-517	3.47 / 3.79 / 3.98	3.37 / 3.78 / 4.0	Y
125	Vanderbilt				
	32 / 36 / 40	508-509 / 515 / 521	3.66 / 3.88 / 3.99	3.59 / 3.88 / 4.0	N
126	Virginia Common Wealth				
	28 / 31 / 35	504 / 508 / 514	3.33 / 3.72 / 3.97	3.22 / 3.69 / 3.97	N
127	Virginia Tech				
	31 / 33 / 37	508 / 511 / 516-517	3.33 / 3.51 / 3.87	3.13 / 3.44 / 3.86	N
128	Wake Forest				
	28 / 33 / 36	508 / 511 / 515	3.36 / 3.72 / 3.95	3.25 / 3.69 / 3.97	N
129	Washington University				
	34 / 38 / 41	512-513 / 518 / 522	3.69 / 3.9 / 4.0	3.63 / 3.91 / 4.0	N
130	Wayne State				
	29 / 32 / 37	505-506 / 509-510 / 516-517	3.5 / 3.85 / 3.97	3.41 / 3.81 / 3.98	Y
131	Western Michigan				
	29 / 32 / 35	505-506 / 509-510 / 514	3.44 / 3.71 / 3.93	3.32 / 3.63 / 3.93	N

#	School				
	MCAT (OLD)	MCAT (NEW)	GPA ALL	GPA S	In-State
132	**West Virginia**				
	26 / 29 / 34	501 / 505-506 / 512-513	3.52 / 3.82 / 3.99	3.42 / 3.77 / 4.0	Y
133	**Wright State**				
	26 / 31 / 35	501 / 508 / 514	3.3 / 3.73 / 3.95	3.17 / 3.65 / 3.98	Y
134	**Yale**				
	32 / 37 / 41	509-510 / 516-517 / 522	3.63 / 3.88 / 3.99	3.55 / 3.88 / 4.0	N

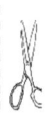

Chart 5: Secondary Application Question Codes

Code	Category
AU	Auto-Biographical / Uniqueness
DE	Diversity Experience
PB	Postbac Experience
CS	Challenging Situations
SS	School Specific
FP	Future Plans
O	Other

Chart 6: Secondary Application Questions

1	**Albany Medical College**
O	1. If you have previously applied to Albany Medical College or another medical school and were not accepted, how have you spent the intervening time?
AU	2. Describe yourself.
O	3. Explain any inconsistencies in your academic performance and/or MCAT scores.
PB	4. Has your college or university, graduate or professional school attendance been interrupted for any reason? If so, explain. Also, explain any gaps in your post-graduate history.
AU	5. Tell us one thing about yourself that would help determine if you should be admitted to our program.
AU	6. Select the most meaningful experience influencing your desire to pursue a career in medicine, explain why, and describe what aspect of that experience best equips you to make an impact in the medical profession.
2	**Albert Einstein**
	If YES, then provide a 100-word explanation
PB	1. I have taken time off between high school and college.
PB	2. I have taken time off during my undergraduate years.
PB	3. I have taken off at least a year since college graduation.
PB	4. I plan to take off this year, after just having graduated, while I apply to medical school.
O	5 -26. Many specific questions about personal history.

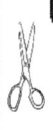

3	**Baylor**
O	1. Indicate any special experiences, unusual factors or other information you feel would be helpful in evaluating you, including, but not limited to, education, employment, extracurricular activities, or prevailing over adversity.

4	**Boston University**
O	1. If you did not go to college directly after high school, please explain.
PB	2. If you are not expecting to go directly to medical school after completing your undergraduate work, please explain.
O	3. If you have spent more than 4 years as an undergraduate, please explain below.
AU	4. Please provide a narrative or timeline to describe any features of your educational history that you think may be of particular interest to us. This is an opportunity to describe learning experiences not be covered in other areas.

5	**Brown (Warren Alpert)**
PB	1. Summarize your activities for the academic year and describe how they are preparing you for a medical career.
DE	2. How will your unique attributes add to the overall diversity of the Alpert Medical School community?
FP	3. What are your aspirations for your medical practice? 15 years in the future: where do you imagine yourself?

6	**Case Western**
CS	1. Describe a significant personal challenge you have faced, one which you feel has helped to shape you as a person. Please include how you got through the experience and what you may have learned about yourself as a result.
AU	2. Describe a research experience, including the question you pursued and how you approached it, your results and interpretation of the results, and most importantly, any thoughts about what this experience meant to you.
AU	3. Did you help to answer a question? Did you help in producing results? Can you interpret those results and explain what they mean? Explain what you learned from your research experience as a whole and what it meant to you.
O	4. If you were working on a small group project and you thought that another student wasn't carrying his/her load, how would you handle it?

7	**Central Michigan**
FP	1. Write a goal focused individual mission statement for your medical career.
SS	2. Please tell us why you are interested in attending the CMU College of Medicine?
DE	3. How do you define diversity, what experience have you had with diversity, and how would you benefit from an environment that embraces diversity?
FP	4. In looking beyond graduation from medical school, please describe what you anticipate will be your most meaningful opportunity as a physician.
O	5. Please provide any additional information that you wish the committee to consider.
SS	6. If out of state, describe any ties that you have to Central Michigan University and/or the state of Michigan.
8	**Columbia**
O	1. Please describe your parents' occupations.
PB	2. If you took time off from your undergraduate studies, please briefly summarize your reasons.
AU	3. In what collegiate extracurricular activities did you engage?
O	4. Describe any work for compensation during college during the year or the summer.
PB	5. If you have graduated from college, please briefly summarize what you have done in the interim.
CS	6. What challenges do you expect to arise from living and working in a complex urban environment? How will you meet them?
9	**Cornell Weill**
PB	1. If you are not attending college during the upcoming academic year, what are your plans?

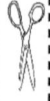

9 Cornell Weill Continued	
SS	2. Please write a brief statement giving your reasons for applying to Weill Cornell Medical College.
CS	3. Please describe a challenge you faced and how you addressed it.
10	**Creighton University**
SS	1. Please state your reasons for applying to Creighton University School of Medicine
FP	2. How will becoming a Creighton-educated physician enable you to achieve your lifetime goals and/or aspirations?
PB	3. Please describe your current activities/employment if you are not currently enrolled as a full-time student.
11	**Dartmouth (Geisel)**
PB	1. Please indicate your plans for the academic year. If in school, please list your courses. If working, let us know something about the nature of your job.
O	2. Please share with us something about yourself that is not addressed elsewhere in your application and which could be helpful to the Admissions Committee.
12	**Drexel University**
PB	1. Give details about any interruption or time away from your education. Detail your activities for each year.
13	**Duke**
AU	1. Describe the community in which you were nurtured or spent the majority of your early development with respect to its demographics. What core values did you receive and how will these translate into the contributions that you hope to make to your community as a medical student and to your career in medicine?
CS	2. What is the most difficult obstacle you have faced? What resources did you marshal to confront it? How did the experience affect you and/or transform your life?

	13 Duke Continued
CS	3. What has been your most humbling experience and how will that experience affect your interactions with your peers and patients?
	4. Essay Pick one optional:
AU	a. Giving back to your community: What is the value of giving back to your community? Is it a more important attribute of a physician than of others performing other roles within a community?
AU	b. How are you misunderstood: What are people most likely to misunderstand about you and why?
CS	c. Toughest feedback: What is the toughest feedback that you ever received? How did you handle it and what did you learn from it?
14	**East Carolina (Brody)**
AU	1. Please use this area to submit a composition which reflects your reasons for desiring to study medicine, future professional aspirations, most significant clinical experience, and also most meaningful non-medical experience.
15	**East Tennessee (Quillen)**
O	The AMCAS application is not designed to capture unique, special, or unusual circumstances. With this in mind, what other information would help the Admissions Committee obtain a more comprehensive picture of your candidacy?
16	**Eastern Virginia**
AU	1. Briefly describe your exposure to medicine.
FP	2. What do you think you will like best about being a physician?
FP	3. What do you think you will like least about being a physician?
FP	4. Describe yourself and your medical career as you see it ten years from now.
SS	5. Please indicate your reasons for applying to EVMS.

17	Emory
PB	1. Please list your entire curriculum plan for the academic year. If you are not currently in school, please briefly describe what you are doing now.
AU	2. Briefly describe your health-related experiences.
SS	3. Briefly describe your interest in Emory.
FP	4. What do you consider to be the role of the physician in the community?
O	5. Include any updates or new information to report since you have submitted your primary application.

18	Florida Atlantic
FP	1. In the event that you are accepted to two or more medicals schools, what factors would be most important in determining which school would be the "best fit" for you.
AU	2. Describe an experience unrelated to science or medicine that you've had in each of the categories. a. A community service experience (unrelated to science or patient care). b. An employment experience (a job you held for pay unrelated to science or medicine). c. A position of responsibility/authority (in which others depended on you for direction). d. A creative endeavor (e.g. art, dance, music, computer programming, website design, writing) e. A situation in which you interacted with individuals who were different from you.
SS	3. Describe any compelling humanitarian reason you have to attend our College of Medicine.

19	Florida International University
PB	1. Whether or not you will be a full-time student, please provide details of your activities for the application year.
SS	2. Given our unique mission, describe how your personal characteristics and values make you a suitable candidate for medicine. How will you contribute to the student body?
CS	3. Describe how you have handled a personal or academic challenge. Focus on what you learned about yourself and how it will help you face possible challenges in medical school.

	19 Florida International University Continued
DE	4. Explain in detail an experience in which you collaborated, worked or were exposed to diverse backgrounds different from your own. Please describe the impact the experience had on you.
AU	5. Give an example when you were part of a team. What was your role in the team? How did you contribute to this task group? How often did you interact with other team members?

20	**Florida State**
AU	1. Indicate your significant travel experiences and include the circumstances.
AU	2. Indicate what you do for fun and diversion (hobbies, special interests, etc.).
AU	3. Identify any of your traits, habits, experiences, or interests that a professor or adviser would not normally know.
AU	4. For both mother and father, give the following: Where they were raised, 4-5 traits that would describe him/her to a stranger, traits you get from him/her, your rapport with him/her, his/her hobbies or interests. Give names, ages and a few brief comments about your brothers and sisters.
FP	5. In what field of medicine do you envision yourself working ten years from now?
O	6. Write a critical analysis of your personal and scholastic qualifications for medicine and professional ambitions.

21	**George Washington University**
O	1. Have you ever been convicted of, plead guilty, or plead no lo contendere to a criminal offense? Have you ever been arrested for a felony or misdemeanor? Did you indicate that you were the recipient of any institutional action on your AMCAS application?
PB	2. For the application cycle, please indicate activities, academics, employment, or other occupations to account for full-time activity (approx. 30-40 hours per week).
AU	3. What is your most significant achievement outside the classroom?
CS DE	4. What makes you a unique individual? What challenges have you faced? How will these factors help you contribute to the diversity of the student body at GW?

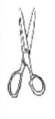

	21 George Washington University Continued
SS	5. What is your specific interest GW? What opportunities would you take advantage of as a student here? Why?
22	**Georgetown University**
DE	1. Describe how any personal characteristics or life experiences will contribute to the diversity of, and bring educational benefits to, our student body.
SS	2. Why have you chosen to apply to Georgetown University School of Medicine, and how do you think your education at Georgetown will prepare you to become a physician for the future?
O	3.Is there any further information that you would like us to be aware of when reviewing your file that you were not able to notate in another section of this or the AMCAS Application?
23	**Harvard**
PB	1. If you have already graduated, briefly summarize your activities since graduation.
O	2. Share any important aspect of your personal background or identity, not addressed elsewhere in the application.
24	**Hofstra North Shore**
PB	1. If you are currently not a matriculated student, please indicate what you have been doing since the time of graduation until now.
O	2. If your undergraduate education was interrupted for any reason, please indicate the reasons, the duration of the interruption, and how you spent your time.
O	3. Please share anything your application does not include, but that you would like to bring to our attention.
25	**Howard University**
DE	1. Have you lived (for three years or more) in communities which are medically underserved, or where the majority of the population is economically and/or educationally disadvantaged?

	25 Howard University Continued
FP	2. After residency, do you plan to practice medicine in an underserved or disadvantaged community?
DE	3. Have you worked (volunteer or paid employment) with medically underserved, economically disadvantaged, and/or educationally disadvantaged populations?
O	4. Are you self-described as a Native American?
O	5. Have you ever been convicted of a felony or misdemeanor in any jurisdiction?
O	6. Please provide below any additional information you believe is important in evaluating your application (e.g. additional coursework, problems with academic record, disadvantaged, etc.)
FP	7. What are you currently doing or what do you plan to do in the next 9-12 months?
FP	8. I am now currently working or plan to work: In Biomedical or Clinical Research? Full or Part-time in medicine or a medical-related field (Nursing, EMT, PA, Office Assistant, etc.)? Full or part-time in a field outside of medicine?
26	**Indiana University**
O	Unknown.
27	**Jefferson Medical College**
O	1. Have you ever been convicted of a crime other than a minor traffic or parking violation? If you answer yes, please provide an explanation in the space provided.
O	2. If there is any additional information you would like to provide, please include it in the box below.
28	**Johns Hopkins**
PB	1. If you have already received your bachelor's degree, please describe what you have been doing since graduation and your plans for the upcoming year.

	28 Johns Hopkins Continued
PB	2. If you interrupted your college education for a semester or longer, please describe that time.
AU	3. List any academic honors or awards you have received since entering college.
AU	4. Briefly describe your single, most rewarding experience.
FP	5. Are there any areas of medicine that are of particular interest to you?
CS	6. Briefly describe a situation where you had to overcome adversity; include lessons learned and how you think it will affect your career as a future physician.
DE	7. Briefly describe a situation where you were not in the majority. What did you learn from this experience?
29	**Loma Linda**
SS	1. Describe the extent and source of your knowledge of Loma Linda University School of Medicine. What makes LLUSM particularly attractive to you? What qualities make you a desirable candidate for admission to LLUSM?
O	2. Discuss how your spiritual experience has influenced your life and how you integrate it.
O	3. What experiences in your life would illustrate your perspective on service to others?
O	4. Please explain integrating a Christian perspective into the practice of medicine as it relates to your personal educational and career goals.
O	5. As a Seventh-day Adventist institution, our lifestyle expectations include abstinence from alcohol, tobacco and illicit drugs/substances in all forms. In the past year, have you used any of these substances? If so, which one(s)?
30	**Loyola (Stritch)**
AU	1. Describe a valuable experience in your personal development. This might be a decision you have made, an achievement of which you are particularly proud of, or a person who has influenced your life.

30 Loyola (Stritch) Continued	
DE	2. Provide in detail an experience of working with individual(s) from diverse background(s). What was the experience? How did it have an impact on you?
CS	3. Describe how you have dealt with a personal or academic challenge. Focus on what you learned about yourself and how it will help you during the challenges you might face in medical school.
O	4. Your patient has a rare disease and would be a great candidate for an experimental new treatment. You are the principal investigator for the research project, and you and your Chair would like to pursue this experiment with the patient. The parents of your patient are adamant against the treatment. How would you handle this situation?
PB	5. If you will not be enrolled as a full-time student during the current academic year, please explain what you will be doing prior to your planned matriculation into medical school.
O	6. Please use this space to bring the information in your AMCAS application up-to-date.
31	**LSU New Orleans**
O	Unknown.
32	**LSU Shreveport**
O	Unknown.
33	**Mayo Medical School**
O	No Essay.
34	**Marshall University (Edwards)**
SS	1. Why did you decide to apply to the Marshall University Joan C. Edwards School of Medicine?
FP	2. Where do you see yourself in 10 years? Where do you want to serve or practice medicine?

	34 Marshall University (Edwards) Continued
PB	3. If you are not presently attending school, indicate your employment or other plans for the time prior to your planned enrollment in medical school.
35	**Medical College Georgia**
CS	1. The Committee strongly encourages you to share unique, personally important, and/or challenging factors in your background. Please discuss how such factors have influenced your goals and preparation for a career in medicine.
FP	2. Please describe the geographical setting in which you think you would most like to practice following medical training.
O	3. Indicate any special experiences, unusual factors or other information you have not already addressed that you feel the Admissions Committee should consider when evaluating your application.
36	**Medical College Wisconsin**
SS	Choose one of the areas from our mission statement and discuss how you will contribute to our mission, both as a medical student and a practicing physician.
37	**Medical University of South Carolina**
O	Unknown.
38	**Meharry Medical College**
SS	1. Why are you applying to Meharry? Focus on school mission: serving the underserved.
39	**Mercer**
SS	1. How do you plan to contribute to healthcare in rural or underserved Georgia?
SS	2. Please describe a service or volunteer activity that you feel best prepared you for the mission of our school?

	39 Mercer Continued
O	3. What ethical dilemmas do you foresee that you might encounter in medical practice in rural and underserved Georgia? Please describe one such incident and how you might resolve it.
AU	4. Would you consider yourself disadvantaged as compared to the 'average' medical school applicant?
AU	5. Please explain other factors that would help them better understand your unique circumstances?
40	**Michigan State**
CS	1. Discuss a time when you stepped out of your comfort zone. What were the challenges? What did you learn?
AU	2. Describe a personally rewarding experience. What did you learn about yourself through this experience?
AU	3. The vast majority of medical school applicants cite their love of science and strong desire to help others as motivation to enter a career in medicine. If you had to choose one more motivating reason, what would it be and why?
O	4. If you could present yourself to the Committee on Admissions, what would you want to make sure they knew about you?
41	**Morehouse**
AU	1. Set forth the key motivational factors in your decision to apply here and any helpful information about yourself.
42	**Mount Sinai (Icahn)**
AU	1. Please tell us about a passion (professional or personal) you have had thus far in your life.
CS	2. Please tell us about a situation in which working with others has been challenging.

43	NY Medical College
O	Unknown.

44	NYU
O	1. If applicable, please comment on significant fluctuations in your academic record not explained elsewhere.
PB	2. If you have taken any time off from your studies, either during or after college, please describe.
SS	3. What unique qualities or experiences do you possess that would contribute specifically here?

4. Please answer only one of the following three questions:

AU	a. The most meaningful achievements are often non-academic in nature. Describe the personal accomplishment that makes you most proud. Why is this important to you?
CS	b. Conflicts arise daily from differences in perspectives, priorities, worldviews, and traditions. Describe a situation in which you found it challenging to remain respectful while facing differences.
CS	c. Describe a situation in which working with a colleague, family member or friend has been challenging. How did you resolve, if at all, the situation as a team and what did you gain from the experience that will benefit you as a future healthcare provider?

45	Northwest Ohio
DE	1. Provide a specific example of how you promoted diversity in your community.
AU	2. How has your view of social justice in medicine been influenced by a specific experience or activity?
FP	3. What physician activity will be most meaningful to you? Provide a specific life experience affirming its meaningfulness.

46	Northwestern
SS	1. Given the distinctive educational philosophy and curriculum at FSM, describe how your personal characteristics and learning style would fit the institution.
CS	2. Describe the coping skills (not problem-solving skills) you use when confronted with difficult situations.
FP	3. Describe your career plans and goals. Be as specific as your current thinking will allow.
PB	4: If you have (or expect to have) a year or more between college graduation and Medical school matriculation, describe your activities and/or plans.
AU	5. If you wish, use this space to provide more detail about your selections about your racial background, sexual identity, and social background and how you would bring diversity to the Northwestern community.
47	**Oakland University**
AU	1. What have you done to make your community a better place?
O	2. Is there anything you want the admissions committee to know about your qualifications for medical school that is not already represented in your application materials?
PB	3. Please explain any gaps in your education, if applicable.
48	**Ohio State**
FP	1. Describe how you would like to contribute to ensuring quality healthcare for all people.
SS	2. Briefly describe how you aspire to further our mission as a medical student or as an alumnus.
49	**Oregon Health & Science University**
AU	1. What experience have you had that has given you insight into the patients you hope to eventually serve?

	49 Oregon Health & Science University Continued
FP	2. What will be your greatest challenge in becoming a physician?
CS	3. Describe a problematic situation working with a person or a group. What did you learn?
AU	4. Describe a time when you did not receive what you felt you deserved, and how you reacted.
AU	5. Give an example of personal feedback that was difficult to receive. How did you respond?
DE	6. Please discuss the diversity that you would bring here and the profession of medicine.
CS	7. While you were growing up, did you experience any adversity? Describe.
50	**Pennsylvania State University**
O	1. Is there a unique aspect of your application that should be considered by the admissions committee?
SS	2. Explain why you decided to apply to Penn State College of Medicine.
AU	3. Please write a short paragraph describing a significant experience you have had working in a team setting.
CS	4. Briefly describe an experience where you had to navigate a complex system to achieve an end. Reflect on the qualities and attributes required by you to achieve success.
51	**Quinnipiac University (Netter)**
FP	1. What medical specialty are you considering? What factors have influenced your decision?
SS	2. How do you see yourself contributing to the learning environment at the Frank H. Netter MD School of Medicine?

	51 Quinnipiac University (Netter) Continued
CS	3. Please answer only two of the questions. a. Describe an experience outside your level of comfort and what lesson(s) you gained from the experience.
AU	b. Describe an occasion when you inspired others.
CS	c. Discuss how you have coped with a setback.
52	**Rosalind Franklin Chicago Medical**
SS	1. Why did you choose to apply to the Chicago Medical School at RFUMS?
DE	2. We encourage you to submit an optional diversity statement that specifically addresses how, if admitted to our program, your admission would contribute to the diversity here.
53	**Rowan University (Cooper)**
SS	1. How is Camden, New Jersey either similar to or different from communities you have experienced? How do you believe that these factors will impact your medical education?
AU	2. In what way have you made an impact or difference to a school, job, organization, or person in your life?
AU	3. As you reflected on what to include in your personal statement to AMCAS, how did you decide which aspects of yourself to highlight?
AU	4. Which undergraduate course taught you the most about yourself? Please explain.
54	**Rush Medical College**
AU	1. Describe personal attributes you possess or life experiences you have had that will enable you to better understand patients with a culture different from your own.
AU	2. Identify community service activities in which you have participated in during the last five years.

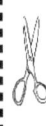

137

	54 Rush Medical College Continued
AU	3. Please describe your most significant achievement outside the classroom.
SS	4. Describe your specific interest in Rush Medical College and what campus opportunities you would most look forward to as a student).
55	**Rutgers University (NJMS)**
O	1. Please discuss any personal characteristics that make you a good fit for medicine, as well as a good fit for us.
SS	2. If your legal residence on your AMCAS application is not NJ, please discuss specific reasons you have applied to NJMS and include connections you may have (if any) to New Jersey.
O	3. Please discuss any additional information you feel is important to your candidacy for medical school.
PB	4. If you are not attending college/university full time as of fall or during the rest of the academic year, please describe your planned activities until from June – August.
56	**Rutgers University (RWJMS)**
O	Unknown.
57	**Saint Louis University**
O	1. Please list year/s of previous applications to this school.
O	2. Is any member of your family a student or graduate of Saint Louis University School of Medicine?
PB	3. Will you be a full-time student for the academic year?
O	4. Do you wish to include any comments, other than your AMCAS personal statement?

	57 Saint Louis University Continued
O	5. Were you ever the recipient of any action by any college for unacceptable academic performance or conduct violations?
58	**Southern Illinois University**
SS	1. In what ways do you believe you would contribute to this mission?
DE	2. Describe a contribution in a teamwork setting; engagement in self-directed and life-long learning and exposure to the small group tutorial process used in a problem-based learning environment.
O	3. Please describe how you feel you have strengthened your credentials since a previous application.
59	**Stanford**
DE	1. The Committee on Admissions strongly encourages you to share unique, personally important, and/or challenging factors in your background. Discuss any factors influencing your goals and preparation for a career in medicine.
FP	2. What do you see as the most likely practice scenario for your future medical career?
FP	3. Choose the single answer that best describes your career goals: Private Practice; Health Policy; Academic Medicine; Public Health; Healthcare Administration
FP	3. Why do you feel you are particularly suited for this practice scenario? What knowledge, skills, and attitudes have you developed that have prepared you for this career path?
SS	4. How will the Stanford curriculum, and specifically the requirement for a scholarly concentration, help your personal career goals?
60	**Stony Brook**
O	1. Many specific questions about your history.
FP	2. Tell us what you anticipate you will be doing professionally 15 years after graduating from medical school and why.

	60 Stony Brook Continued
PB	3. Explain what you have done or plan to do during the gap period and why.
CS	4. Describe an obstacle you've overcome and how it has defined you.
61	**SUNY Downstate**
PB	1. If there were periods longer than 3 months, from the time you graduated from high school to now, when you were not employed full-time or in college full-time, please briefly describe your activities.
PB	2. If you are not attending college full time as of September, please describe your activities for the period September to July. Please enter none if there are none.
SS	3. If you are not from the 5 boroughs of New York City, describe what personal experiences prepare you to live and study in New York City, and what will be your personal support system?
SS	4. Explain any specific reason why you wish to attend SUNY Downstate or a medical school in New York City.
62	**SUNY Upstate**
O	Unknown.
63	**Temple**
SS	1. What is the nature of your special interest in Temple University School of Medicine?
SS	2. How do you anticipate contributing to the TUSM community?
SS	3. If you indicated one of our clinical campuses as your first choice, describe the nature of your interest.
FP	4. What are your plans for the current year?

64	Texas A&M
DE	1. Describe any experiences making you sensitive or appreciative of other cultures or the human condition.
AU	2. Discuss activities or personal attributes that demonstrate your understanding of our honor code.
O	3. Describe any circumstances indicative of some hardship.
FP	4. List the area (or areas) of medicine that appeals to you and briefly explain.
65	Texas Tech (El Paso)
DE	1. Recognizing the components of the mission and location on the US/Mexico border, describe your interest.
AU	2. Describe how someone influenced your aspirations to obtain a medical degree.
AU	3. Describe past experiences or personal attributes that reflect your affinity with the TTUSHC is honor code.
CS	4. Describe any personal experiences or disadvantage and its significance to your pursuit of a medical degree.
66	Commonwealth Medical College
O	1. Imagine that you are a family physician and are seeing a 15-year-old girl for menstrual cramps. Her mother has accompanied her for this visit. When you examine the patient without her mother present, she tells you that she is sexually active. She begs you not to tell her mother because of her family's strong values against teen sex. Discuss your next steps.
67	Tufts
O	1. Do you wish to include any comments to the Admissions Committee?
DE	2. Do you consider yourself a person who would contribute to the diversity of the student body of Tufts?

	67 Tufts Continued
PB	3. Did you take any leaves of absence or significant breaks from your undergraduate education?
O	4. Is any member of your family a graduate of TUSM or a current member of our faculty?
68	**Tulane**
SS	1. Briefly describe the reasons for your interest in Tulane University School of Medicine.
AU	2. What was the single most meaningful volunteer experience you have had?
AU	3. List any leadership positions, in clubs or organizations, you may have held during college.
AU	4. Please list your hobbies and major non-academic interests (e.g. athletics, art, music, items you collect, genre or favorite author reading material).
69	**Uniformed Services University**
SS	1. Please describe your motivation to learn and practice medicine with the U.S. military medical corps and/or the U.S. Public Health Service.
SS	2. Please describe what in your research about our school and/or in your personal or family background attracts you to our institution's unique mission and approach.
DE	3. Please describe a special quality or experience that will help you relate to our unique population and that will strengthen your class if admitted to "America's Medical School.
70	**University of Alabama**
FP	1. Where do you see yourself in your medical career fifteen to twenty years from now?
O	2. Please share any not-included information you want us to know about you.

71	**University of Arizona (Tucson)**
AU	1. Please share a meaningful experience you have had working or volunteering in the health profession. What did you learn from this as it relates to becoming a physician?
CS	2. Discuss a time in your life in which you have failed at something other than an academic experience. How did you confront the failure and what did you learn from it?
FP	3. A key part of our mission is to train physicians to address healthcare disparities in the United States. What role will you play in addressing healthcare disparities in the United States?
DE	4. Describe the effect that your experiences engaging diversity have had on your own growth and development. Provide an example and describe how it will impact your career in the medical profession.
72	**University of Arizona (Phoenix)**
O	1. Have you previously applied to The University of Arizona College of Medicine-Phoenix? Why do you feel you are a stronger applicant this year?
SS	2. After learning more about our mission and values as a medical school, share how you fit within the AU Phoenix Med culture.
PB	3. Elaborate on what has occurred in the last 12-18 months that has influenced your goal and preparation for a career in medicine.
CS	4. What unique or challenging factors in your background (childhood/adulthood) have enhanced your character?
O	5. What is important to you that you want to make sure the Admissions Committee knows about you that is not already included in your application?
73	**University of Arkansas**
O	Unknown.
74	**University Buffalo**
O	Unknown.

75	**UC Davis**
O	1. Discuss any elements of your application that you feel might be concerning to the Admissions Committee.
SS	2. How will your family, community, academic, work or other life experiences enhance UC Davis?
CS	3. What do you foresee as challenges in medical school and your future career?
PB	4. What have you been doing since submitting your application? Include contact references.
O	5. If applicable tell us why you would like to be considered for the Rural-PRIME program. B. Please describe your experiences working with underserved communities. C. What are your future plans to practice in a rural underserved community?
O	6. If you would like to be considered for Davis ACE-PC, please tell us what attributes or experiences would make you a good fit for the program. If you are not interested, please insert "Not Applicable".
SS	7. Please tell us about your ties to the San Joaquin Valley. B. Please describe an experience where you learned about a challenge in the San Joaquin Valley. C. After you complete your medical training, where do you intend to practice and why?
O	8. If interested in the PST, describe your experience, qualifications, and goals.
76	**UC Irvine**
AU	1. What personal accomplishment are you most proud of and why?
CS	2. Please describe to the Admissions Committee a challenge you have overcome and what you learned about yourself.
PB	3. Please clarify your activities since receiving your undergraduate degree.
77	**UCLA**
AU	1. Describe involvement in the one most important non-academic activity that has been important in your life.

	77 UCLA Continued
AU	2. What has been the one most unique leadership, entrepreneurial, or creative activity in which you participated?
AU	3. What has been the one most important volunteer work you have done and why was it meaningful?
AU	4. What is the one most important honor you have received? Why do you view this as important?
AU	5. What has been your most scholarly project (thesis, research or field of study in basic or clinical science or in the humanities)? Describe one and give the number of hours, dates and advisor.
CS	6. Describe a problem in your life. Include how you dealt with it and how it influenced your growth.
O	7. List major paid work experience during (or since) college. Give dates, description, and approximate hours.
O	8. If there is any hardship to which you would like the committee to give special attention in evaluating your application, then check the box labeled 'Hardship' and briefly explain why.
FP	9. Where do you see yourself in 10 years? What experiences have led you to this goal?
78	**UC Riverside**
AU	1. Describe the single MOST important non-academic activity in your life and explain its significance.
AU	2. What has been your single MOST unique leadership, entrepreneurial, or creative activity?
AU	3. What has been the single MOST important volunteer work you have done and why was it meaningful?
AU	4. What is the MOST important honor (one) you have received? Why do you view this as important?
AU	5. What has been your MOST scholarly project (thesis, research, or field of study in basic or clinical sciences or in the humanities)? Describe one and give the number of hours, dates, and advisor(s).

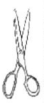

	78 UC Riverside Continued
CS	6. Describe a major problem at some time in your life, how you dealt with it and how it influenced you.
O	7. Is there any specific hardship to which you would like the committee to know?
FP	8. Where do you see yourself in 10 years? What experiences have led you to this goal?
AU	9. What is the most important healthcare issue confronting disadvantaged communities and what would be your first steps to address this issue?
O	10. You may use this space to provide any further information you may want us to consider in addition to the personal statement.
79	**UC San Diego**
AU	1. This should be a true autobiographical statement with family, childhood, primary and secondary school years, undergraduate years, what you've done since completing your bachelor's degree, and the motivational factors which led you to a career in medicine including any disadvantages or obstacles which might put your accomplishments into context.
80	**UC San Francisco**
O	1. If you wish to update or expand upon your activities, you may provide additional information below.
81	**University of Central Florida**
PB	1. If you do not expect to spend the academic year enrolled in an academic program, please explain.
O	2. Please provide details regarding academic difficulties, grades below B minus or course withdrawals.
AU	3. Please provide a short essay to help us understand who you are.

82	University of Chicago (Pritzker)
DE	1. In particular, our mission highlights the value placed on diversity as we regard diversity as essential for educational excellence. Please write an essay on how you would enhance diversity and advance the mission.
CS	2. Tell us about a difficult or challenging situation you have encountered and how you dealt with it.
O	3. Additional Information. Please feel free to use this space to convey any additional information.
83	University of Cincinnati
O	1. Were you ever the recipient of an institutional action? If yes, please explain.
O	2. Have you ever participated in a pre-conviction program or been convicted of, pled guilty, or no contest to a felony and/or criminal offense? If yes, please explain.
O	3. Have you been convicted of or pled guilty or no contest to, any moving traffic violations (moving violations include speeding tickets)? If yes, please explain.
O	4. Have you ever matriculated at or attended any medical school as a candidate for the MD degree? If yes, please explain.
PB	5. If you are NOT currently enrolled in a degree-granting program, please briefly describe your major activities, not listed on AMCAS.
84	University of Colorado
AU	1. Write about things important to your development or challenging to you on your path to a career in medicine. Explain how these have influenced your goals and preparation this career. Explain the "fit" between your experiences and goals and the University of Colorado School of Medicine.
85	University of Connecticut
AU	1. Highlight your experiences in the healthcare field. What insights have you gained about potential problems you will face as a physician?
CS	2. Describe the activity from which you gained the greatest personal benefit and insight.

	85 University of Connecticut Continued
SS	3. How will we best serve your needs of becoming a physician or physician-scientist?

86	**University of Florida**
PB	1. If you are not a full-time student during this application cycle, detail your current and planned activities.
O	2. Are you more of an extrovert or an introvert and how will this impact how you learn to communicate with patients and colleagues?
AU	3. Consider three areas of integrity: personal, professional, and intellectual. Using an example, describe how these areas may be interrelated. Include why the connection between these areas is significant.
SS	4. Explain any ties to Florida.

87	**University of Hawaii**
AU	1. Describe the important experience(s) that began the process that motivated you to enter a medical career.
SS	2 Explain why you are applying to the University of Hawaii John A. Burns School of Medicine.

88	**University of Illinois**
O	1. Describe a situation in which you were really stressed. Detail your reaction(s), and the effect. If this situation, or a similar one, were to happen again, how would you handle it?
AU	2. Describe a hobby or activity other than something in medicine, in which you have a keen interest. Why?
CS	3. Describe any advantages and/or complications you encountered during your progression in education. Please include any noteworthy achievements and/or obstacles.

89	**University of Iowa**
SS	1. Please explain your reasons for applying to the Carver College of Medicine.
DE	2. Describe any unique personal characteristics and obstacles you may have overcome that will contribute to the diversity of, and bring educational benefits to, the entering class.
AU	3. Please list and provide a brief description of medically related experiences (paid or volunteer) in which you have participated over the past 5 years.
PB	4. Please indicate what you will be doing from now to the start of medical school.
90	**University of Kansas**
AU	1. What experiences have led to your decision to become a physician?
AU	2. Describe examples of leadership experience in which you have significantly influenced others, helped resolve disputes or contributed to group efforts over time.
AU	3. Describe any of your special interests and how you have developed knowledge in these areas. Give examples of your creativity in the ability to see alternatives; to take diverse perspectives; to develop varied or original ideas, or the willingness to try new things.
CS	4. Describe the most significant challenge you have faced and the steps you have taken to address it.
AU	5. Give an example of what you have done to make your community a better place to live.
CS	6. Describe your experiences facing or witnessing discrimination. Tell how you responded and what you learned from these experiences and how they have prepared you for your future in medicine.
DE	7. What special life experiences and/or characteristics would you bring to KU School of Medicine?
AU	8. What do you do for fun?
SS	9. If you are not a Kansas resident, what is your specific interest in applying here?

91	**University of Kentucky**
AU	1. How would you describe your ability to use unscheduled time during the day for learning?
AU	2. What competencies and qualities should a physician possess for practice in the 21st century?
AU	3. Describe the most significant community service activity in which you have participated and its effect.
AU	4. Describe an experience or situation which made you feel grateful.
FB	5. In providing patient care, should physicians maintain emotional distance or empathize with patients' emotional states? As a physician, how would you deal with your own emotions?
AU	6. Describe a situation in your undergraduate education when you felt alive and engaged in learning.
AU	7. Please share unique, personally important, and/or challenging facts in your background. Please discuss how such factors have influenced your goals and preparation for a career in medicine.
92	**University of Louisville**
SS	1. If you are an out of state student, please explain your interest in attending here.
AU	2. Please discuss your research experience, including any publications and/or curriculum vitae.
AU	3. What determined your choice of college(s)?
93	**University of Maryland**
AU	1. Briefly describe your most important exposure to clinical medicine.
AU	2. Briefly describe your most satisfying experience related to community service.

93	**93 University of Maryland Continued**
AU	3. What does it mean to you to enter into a profession?
94	**University of Massachusetts**
O	Unknown.
95	**University of Miami**
AU	1. Describe the clinical experience that has most significantly influenced your decision to study medicine.
SS	2. Why have you selected the U of Miami for your medical education? Please be as specific as possible.
96	**University of Michigan**
AU	1. Tell us something you are passionate about and why.
SS	2. What would you as an individual bring to our medical school community?
AU	3. Please list three areas of interest (e.g., symphony orchestra, drawing/painting/ceramics, research in a specific area, joint degrees, athletic interests/running/softball, ballroom dance, Spanish language study, international travel/work/study, etc.) you would like to pursue while at Michigan.
AU	4. We would like to know one fun fact about you. This may be shared with other applicants. Please answer the following question with up to four words: "Most people don't know that I can... "
97	**University of Minnesota**
SS	1. In what ways do you fit the goals of this school?
AU	2. How familiar are you with life in a rural setting or the American Indian community?

	97 University of Minnesota Continued
O	3. What are some professional and personal advantages /disadvantages of a rural family medicine practice?
AU	4. How have you familiarized yourself with the field of medicine?
AU	5. How have your volunteer experiences influenced your life goals?
FP	6. Briefly describe your career plans in the event that you do not attend medical school.
CS	7. Have you ever struggled with being honest and compassionate at the same time? Describe the situation, the struggles and, if there was one, the resolution.
AU	8. Describe an experience you have had working in a team (other than a sports team), what role you played, and your comfort level with that role.
O	9. What does lifelong learning mean to you?
AU	10. What are your recreational and leisure activities?
CS	11. Medical school can be stressful. What coping skills have you used in the past to deal with stressful situations?
98	**University of Mississippi**
O	Unknown.
99	**University of Missouri-Columbia**
O	1. Please describe any element within your candidacy not fully addressed on the AMCAS application.
SS	2. Please outline how you might add to the overall diversity here and the practice of medicine.

100		University Missouri Kansas City
O	Unknown.	

101		University Nebraska
O	Unknown.	

102		University of Nevada
O	Unknown.	

103		University of New Mexico
SS	1. What would you as an individual bring to UNM medical community?	
AU	2. Please describe the unique path that has led you to medicine as well as any obstacles or adversity that you had to overcome in achieving this goal. How will this experience affect your career as a physician?	
FP	3. What do you see as the most significant issues the medical profession will face in the next 20 years, and what are some potential solutions for these problems?	
FP	4. Once you become a physician, how do you foresee yourself helping to address the healthcare challenges that affect communities in the State of New Mexico?	

104		University of North Carolina
O	Unknown	

105		University of North Dakota
O	Unknown	

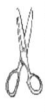

106	**University of Oklahoma**
O	Unknown

107	**University of Pennsylvania (Raymond Ruth Perelman)**
AU	1. Have you been nominated for or received an award from any state, regional or national organization?
PB	2. Have you taken or are you planning to take time off between college graduation and medical school matriculation?
AU	3. Have you participated in any global activities outside of the U.S. prior to submitting your application?
O	4. Are there any special, unique, personal, or challenging circumstances you would like to share?
SS	5. Please explain your reasons for applying to the Perelman School of Medicine.

108	**University of Pittsburgh**
CS	1. Tell us about a challenging problem you faced and how you resolved it
DE	2. How would you enrich/enliven the UPSOM community? The essay should discuss material that is not included in the rest of your application.

109	**University of Rochester**
O	Unknown.

110	**University of South Alabama**
FP	1. Although interests may change, what areas of medicine are you primarily interested in at the present time?

	110 University of South Alabama Continued
DE	2. Please share life experiences that you may have had and/or important factors in your background that illustrate your readiness for practicing medicine in a multicultural society.
111	**University South Carolina Greenville**
O	Unknown.
112	**University of South Carolina**
FP	1. What are your medical practice goals?
AU	2. Does this application represent a career change? If so, please describe your most recent career.
PB	3. If it has been more than six months since you completed your bachelor's degree, please describe your employment status since that time.
FP	4. What areas of medicine are you interested in at this time, or what areas do you plan to pursue?
FP	5. In what region of the country do you want to practice medicine? Why?
AU	6. Do you have any accomplishments or experiences that make you a unique applicant?
113	**University of South Dakota (Sanford)**
SS	1. Please explain how your experiences and long-term goals would help meet the school's mission.
SS	2. Explain how your background and experiences with diversity will bring value here.
FP	3. Describe how your experiences in healthcare or social care activities will help you be a good physician.

	113 University of South Dakota (Sanford) Continued
CS	4. Briefly describe a crisis or significant challenge in your life, how you have worked through the crisis or challenge, and what you have learned from this experience.
FP	5. What are your career plans in the event that you are not admitted to a medical school this year?
114	**University of South Florida**
FP	1. How would the USF'S Scholarly Concentrations Program help your personal career goals?
AU	2. Describe a time in your life when you felt you were "at your best." Why did you choose this event, and how does it reflect your potential as a physician?
AU	3. Who is the best leader you have known in your life? Explain.
DE	4. How do you feel your particular experiences, interests, and passions will add to the strength and diversity of the USF class and ultimately to the field of medicine?
FP	5. Describe your ideas about how the medical profession can best respond to disparities in healthcare.
115	**USC**
AU	1. What is the most fun you've had in the last year?
AU	2. What is the most beautiful sight you've ever seen?
FP	3. If you couldn`t be a health professional, what occupation would you choose?
AU	4. If you could give yourself a nickname, what would it be?
FP	5. If you had enormous wealth, how would you allocate your charitable donations?

115 USC Continued	
AU	6. What aspect of the preparation for becoming a physician did you find most challenging?
DE	7. Have you indicated that you represent a group that is underrepresented in medicine? If so, please explain.
FP	8. How will you be remembered by your medical school classmates 50 years from now?
O	9. Have you ever applied, been accepted, or matriculated to any medical school? If yes, explain.
116	**University Tennessee**
O	Unknown.
117	**University Texas Medical Branch**
O	Unknown.
118	**University Texas Southwestern**
FP	1. Many specific questions about your interests and future plans.
FP	2. Describe the setting in which you envision conducting your medical career.
119	**University of Toledo**
O	1. Briefly discuss any extenuating circumstances which you feel are pertinent to your application.
SS	2. Essay: Please discuss a life experience in which you feel you demonstrated cultural competence.

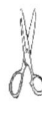

120	**University of Utah**
O	Unknown.

121	**University Vermont**
O	1. Add any additional information.
SS	2. How might you contribute to the overall diversity of the UVM COM community?

122	**University of Virginia**
SS	1. Why are you interested in attending the here? What factors are most important to you in a medical school?
DE	2. How will you contribute to the diversity of your medical school class here?
CS	3. Describe a situation which you found challenging. How did you manage it?

123	**University of Washington**
AU	1. Provide an autobiographical statement.
AU	2. Provide other personal comments or publications.
AU	3. How have your experiences prepared you to be a physician?
DE	4. What perspectives or experiences do you bring that would enrich the class?
CS	5. What obstacles have you experienced and how have you overcome them?

124	**University of Wisconsin**
AU	1. Provide a chronological history of your activities from the time you completed high school to the present.
AU	2. Explain what makes you exceptional and why you will become an outstanding physician.

125	**Vanderbilt**
AU	1. Write a brief autobiography.
CS	2. Please discuss a challenging situation or obstacle you have faced in the past. Why was it challenging? How did you handle it? Knowing what you know now, would you do anything differently? What did you learn?

126	**Virginia Commonwealth**
O	1. A family member or friend comes to you to discuss a curable cancer for which they are considering alternative medicine options. What would be your next steps?

127	**Virginia Tech**
O	Unknown.

128	**Wake Forest**
DE	1. Wake Forest School of Medicine believes that the quality of an educational experience depends in part on the differences in backgrounds, experiences, and perspectives of the students who comprise each class. How will you contribute to the diversity of your medical school class?
CS	2. What obstacles or challenges have you experienced and how have you dealt with them?
AU	3. The Association of American Medical Colleges (AAMC) lists 14 entry-level core competencies for medical school applicants: Please pick ONE of the competencies and describe how your background and experiences highlight the competency and prepares you for medical school.
PB	4. If you have already received your bachelor's degree, please describe what you have been doing since graduation and your plans for the upcoming year.

	128 Wake Forest Continued
O	5. If you are a re-applicant, please describe if you have made any significant changes or improvements from your previous application.
SS	6. Describe any connection you have to Wake Forest School of Medicine, Wake Forest University, Winston-Salem, or North Carolina.
129	**Washington University**
O	1. Do you have unique experiences or obstacles that you have overcome that were not covered in your application about which you would like to inform our Admissions Committee?
CS	2. Describe a time or situation where you have been unsuccessful or failed.
PB	3. If you have already completed your education, if your college or graduate education was interrupted, or if you do not plan to be a full-time student during the current year, describe in chronological order your activities during the time(s) when you were not enrolled as a full-time student.
130	**Wayne State**
O	Unknown.
131	**Western Michigan**
SS	1. Describe why you wish to enroll at Western Michigan.
AU	2. Describe what you bring to the practice of medicine - your values, skills, talents, and life experiences - and how you add to the cultural, ethnic, and socioeconomic diversity of the medical profession
132	**West Virginia**
FP	1. Imagine a world in which illness and injury do not exist. All hospitals and medical schools have closed because there is no longer a need. What would you choose to do with your life in such a world?

132	**132 West Virginia Continued**
CS	2. Describe a time when you failed despite your best efforts. How would you handle it differently now?
AU	3. Other than a family member, who has been the most influential person in your life and why?
O	4. You are the Chair of the Committee on Admissions: What would you consider to be the most important feature or component of a candidate's application?
133	**Wright State**
O	Unknown.
134	**Yale**
SS	1. Please use this space to write an essay in which you discuss your interest in Yale School of Medicine.
O	2. This section should be used to bring to the attention of the Admissions Committee any information not previously discussed throughout your Yale Secondary Application.

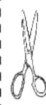

Chart 7: Practice Interview Questions

PERSONAL CHARACTERISTIC QUESTIONS

Personal Background

1. Explain your relationship with your family.

2. Explain your childhood and present living conditions.

3. Explain what you do with your time when not at work or school.

4. Explain what you have been doing since you graduated.

5. Explain how your background will affect your abilities as a physician.

Individual Characteristics

1. Who are you? If you were a cookie, what type would you be? What type of animal would you be? What kind of superhero would you be?

2. How would your teammates or friends describe you? Why?

3. How would your professors or references describe you? Why?

4. How would you describe your personality? If you could change one aspect of yourself, what would it be and why?

5. What are your greatest strengths? Why?

6. What are your greatest weaknesses? Why?

7. What one aspect of your personality would you change if you could?

8. What non-science courses did you enjoy the most? Why?

9. What was your favorite college course? Why?

10. What has been the best thing to occur your life? Explain.

Thought Processes

1. Explain your decision-making process.

2. Explain your stress management process.

3. Explain a time when you demonstrated initiative.

4. Who has most influenced your life so far and why?

5. Who has been the most influential person in the last 100 years? Why?

6. What book have you read for pleasure lately? Why did you select it? Did you like it?

7. What newspapers, magazines, or journals do you read on a regular basis?

8. What section of the newspaper or news do you read first?

9. What would your decision criteria be if you were accepted by multiple schools?

10. What else would you like us to know before you leave today?

Acquired Activities

1. Explain a situation when you were working in a diverse environment. What did you learn?

2. Explain a situation when you were working on a team. What did you learn?

3. Explain a situation when you faced conflict with someone. What did you learn?

4. Explain a situation in which you were criticized unfairly. What did you learn?

5. Explain any extra-curricular activities you participated in. What did you learn?

6. Explain what you have done to keep in touch with your community's needs.

7. Explain your most memorable accomplishment in your college career thus far.

8. Explain any medical exposure you have had and its influence on your decision to be a physician.

9. Explain any volunteer experience you have had and its influence on your decision to be a physician.

10. Explain any experiences you have had making you a good candidate for medical school.

Overcoming Adversity

1. Explain a negative teamwork experience and what you learned.

2. Explain a stressful situation and what you learned.

3. Explain a conflict with another person and how it was resolved.

4. Explain a situation when you were criticized unfairly and how it was resolved.

5. Explain a failure and what you learned.

6. Explain a situation in which you felt like you didn't belong and what you learned.

7. Explain a bias you have overcome in your own life and what you learned.

8. Explain the worst thing to occur in your life and what you learned.

9. Explain something in your life you wish you had done differently.

10. Explain what you will do if you do not get admitted to a medical school this cycle.

HEALTHCARE ISSUES

You

1. What is the purpose of medical school?

2. What qualities do you look for in a physician?

3. What are your goals for your medical career?

4. What are the negative aspects of being a physician?

5. What are the rewarding aspects of being a physician?

6. What will you find most difficult about medical school?

7. What is your alternate career path?

8. Why have you chosen medicine to help others instead of social work?

9. Why do you think so many people want to be doctors?

10. Why have you chosen medicine as your career?

You Continued

11. How do you handle any personal problems? Whom do you talk with?

12. How do you think your personal background will affect your medical practice?

13. How could you affect the healthcare system?

14. How will you handle blood and gore?

15. How do you really know that after medical school in 4 years, you'll still want to be a doctor, especially when so many current physicians are unhappy?

Community

1. What community do you most identify with? What are its medical needs?

2. How does your role as a physician fit in with your role as a community member? How do you anticipate fulfilling community needs?

3. How can physicians help the community with social problems like teen pregnancy?

4. Should medical school students receiving federal loans spend time practicing medicine in a rural area or inner city to give society back something in return?

5. Would you practice in the inner city? What do you think happens to people who practice medicine there (attitude changes, etc.)?

World

1. How would you describe the medical profession? Be specific.

2. How do you see the field of medicine changing in the next ten years? How do you see yourself fitting into those changes?

3. Explain your views on the current state of medicine and the changes taking place currently.

4. Explain your views on the most pressing health issue in America today.

5. Explain your views on the Affordable Care Act and how it would affect the physician and the patient.

6. Explain your views on the biggest social problem in the world today and how it affects medicine.

7. Explain your views on the most pressing health issue in the world today.

8. Explain your views on euthanasia.

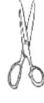

World Continued

9. Explain your views on cloning and who should or shouldn't be cloned.

10 Explain your views on the global refugee crisis.

MEDICAL SCENARIOS

1. If it were 15 years from today, what would your medical career and personal life look like?

2. If you have the choice of giving a transplant to a successful elderly member of the community or a 20-year old drug addict, how do you choose?

3. If there were an accident on the road, would you stop and help the victims, knowing that you doing so might lead to a malpractice claim against you?

4. If a patient told you he/she wanted to commit suicide, what would you do?

5. If your patient had been in an accident and needed a blood transfusion but stated such action was against her religion, what would you do?

6. If your patient requested an abortion, what would you do?

7. If you were treating a patient in the emergency room and he/she wanted to leave against medical advice, what would you do?

8. If you suspect a colleague, another doctor, of abusing drugs, what would you do?

9. If your supervisor asked you to lie to a patient for his/her own good, what would you do?

10. If a colleague wanted you to keep a medical error they made a secret from a patient, what would you do?

SCHOOL SPECIFICS

1. Why did you apply to this school?

2. Why is our medical school a good fit for you?

3. Why should this school pick you over all the other applicants we have to choose from?

4. What do you have to offer to this school?

5. What programs in our school are you interested in?

SCHOOL SPECIFICS CONTINUED

6. What is your opinion of our medical school's curriculum?

7. What other schools have you applied to? Why those?

8. Where does our school stand in your school preferences?

9. How will you be a positive factor in our medical program?

10. How do you plan to finance your medical school education?

YOUR QUESTIONS

1. What kind of opportunities exists for students to design, conduct, and publish research?

2. What kind of counseling (academic, personal, financial, career, etc.) is available to students?

3. What kind of mentors or advisors are available for students?

4. What type of clinical sites is available or required for clerkships?

5. What kind of medical school endowments or financial aid does the school offer?

6. What kind of guidance toward debt management does the school offer?

7. What kind of opportunities for community service does the school offer?

8. How much flexibility exists with coursework during the pre-clinical and clinical years?

9. How are students evaluated academically?

10. How are clinical evaluations performed?

11. Your Personalized Question?

12. Your Personalized Question?

13. Your Personalized Question?

14. Your Personalized Question?

15. Your Personalized Question?

Chart 8: Enlarged Process Timeline

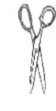

TIMELINE FOR MEDICAL SCHOOL APPLICATION CYCLE

MARCH — MAY	MAY — JUNE	JUNE — JULY	JULY — SEP	SEP — FEB	FEB — APRIL
BE READY	**PREPARE PRIMARY**	**PREPARE SECONDARY**	**PREPARE INTERVIEW**	**ATTEND INTERVIEWS**	**BE SUCCESSFUL**
Acquired ✓ MCAT ✓ Bachelor's ✓ Volunteer ✓ Research	Prepare ✓ Rec Letters ✓ Essay ✓ Activities Choose ✓ Safeties ✓ Standards ✓ Stretches	Plan Responses ✓ AU ✓ DE ✓ PA ✓ CS ✓ FP ✓ SS ✓ O	Plan ✓ Responses ✓ Look ✓ Travel	Complete ✓ Practice ✓ Perform	Choose ✓ Stress ✓ Program ✓ Finances ✓ Environment ✓ Lifestyle

You can get into medical school!!

Coleman's Classroom

Interested in getting help with your medical school application process?

Mrs. C specializes in the written aspects of the primary and secondary application.

If you would like additional information or have any questions or comments, you can reach her on Facebook at www.facebook.com/medicalschoolapplication or by email at classroom@clmn.net.